# ENVISIONING MEDICINE IN THE FUTURE
## With a Universal Patient Medical Record

MICHAEL R. MCGUIRE
(michaelrichardmcguire@gmail.com)

On the cover, the painting "Cortez" by Bayard M. Hedrick

**MCGUIRE PUBLISHING**

MICHAEL R. MCGUIRE
ENVISIONING MEDICINE
IN THE FUTURE
All rights reserved.

No part of this publication may be reproduced, distributed, or transmitted in any form or by any means, including photocopying, recording, or other electronic or mechanical methods, without the prior written permission of the publisher, except in the case of brief quotations embodied in critical reviews and certain other non-commercial uses permitted by copyright law.

MICHAEL R. MCGUIRE

Printed in the United States of America
First Printing 2020
Second Edition 2024
Third Edition 2025

10 9 8 7 6 5 4 3 2 1

# ENVISIONING MEDICINE
IN THE FUTURE

# Table of Contents

*Preface i*

1. *Problems with Current Medicine 1*
2. *The Need for a Complete Patient Medical Record 5*
3. *Electronic Medical Record Systems (EMRs) 7*
4. *Medical Records Within EMRs (Source Documents) 9*
5. *A Clinical Summary 11*
6. *Proposed New Infrastructure for Sharing Patient Medical Information 15*
7. *An Overview of Other Envisioned Future Changes 17*
    *Commercial Ancillary Service Ordering 17*
    *Significant Health Problems for a Patient 17*
    *Extended Care and Increased Physician Responsibility for Care 18*
    *Physicians Working Together in Care 18*
    *Care Across Medical Organizations 19*
    *Transferring Care Between Medical Organizations 19*
    *Order Checking 19*
    *Overall Management of a Patient's Medications 20*
    *Quality-of-Life Used in Care Evaluation 20*
    *Improved End-of-Life Decisions 20*
    *Keeping Patients Well 20*
    *Genetics and the Genome and Other Biomarkers 20*
    *Relatives Sharing Genetic Information 21*
    *Early Treatment 21*
    *Optimizing Physician Time 21*
    *Researching Best Care and Prognoses 22*
    *Accountability 22*
    *Patient Care in Rural Areas 22*

*Public Health* 22
*Confirmed Diagnoses* 23
*Patient Ability to See and Audit the UPMR* 23
*Handling Complicated Medical Problems* 23
Increased Use of Artificial Intelligence 24

**8. Commercial Ancillary Services and Order Checking 25**

**9. Physicians as Story Tellers: Significant Health Problems and Disease Histories 27**

**10. The Three C's 35**

**11. Virtual Organizations 41**

**12. Medication Management 47**

**13. Quality of Life and Other Outcome Measures 51**

**14. Improved End-of-Life Care 57**

**15. Prevention and Self-Care Checklists 61**

**16. Prevention and Health Psychologists 65**

**17. Genetic Information, the Microbiome and Other Biomarkers 69**

**18. Selectively Sharing Genetic Information 73**

**19. Early Treatment Diseases 75**

**20. Optimizing Physician Time Through Scheduling 77**

**21. Research 83**

**22. Population Research: Prognoses and Selection of Interventions 87**

    21.1    Determining if a Medical Intervention is Beneficial 87

21.2   Predicting Typical Results of an Intervention for Similar Patients 90

21.3   Determining the Probability of a Future Outcome 93

21.4   Selecting the Best Intervention 93

21.5   Recovery from a Procedure or Injury 94

21.6   Ad Hoc Studies 94

23. Population Research: Accountability 95

24. Complicated Medical Problems 97

25. Current Emerging Medical Ideas 101

26. Revolutionizing Rural Medicine 103

27. Public Health 107

28. Confirmed Diagnoses 109

29. Patient Mirrored UPMR Access, Auditing and Data Analysis 111

30. Increased Use of Artificial Intelligence 113

31. Precision medicine 119

32. Searching for a Medical Service 121

33. A Projected Example of Precision medicine in the Future 125

34. Design Choices, Alternatives and General Issues 129

35. Where to Next? 133

Glossary 135

References 151

# Preface

This book was written in the tradition of Hugo Gernback, who coined the term "science fiction" and predicted the future in magazine articles in the 1920's, including forecasts of color TV, air conditioning, greater life span, conquering tuberculosis, and fast air travel between New York and Paris (Novak, 2012). These early works of science fiction were not written as fantasies but to predict what science and technology would be like in the coming years.

This book is my vision of what medicine could be like in the future, correcting some of its current failings and accounting for predicted changes to medicine.

There are clear failings in the way medicine functions today. The most obvious is that there is no complete patient medical record, and often when a patient comes in for care, no medical record is readily available to the physician; this despite the fact that there may be one, or there may be many, each of which is likely to have somewhat different medical information.

Medicine itself will change soon. There will be more diagnostic information about the patient, including that at the cellular and genetic level, as well as the tissue level which is the case today.

This additional cellular and genetic information may result in more detailed diagnoses and treatments, although there are some examples today of these more detailed diagnoses (e.g., estrogen-positive and progesterone-positive breast cancer rather than just breast cancer).

Because of the greater number of diagnosis and treatment possibilities, medicine will become even more specialized and thus there is a greater likelihood of a diagnosis or treatment occurring in a medical organization outside the patient's normal one.

This will require greater coordination between physicians in different healthcare institutions than occurs today.

Medicine in the future will also be more data-driven, requiring more and consistent data to be captured. These data will enable patient care to be evaluated and provide more accurate prognoses.

Taking care of current failings and accounting for the new ways in which medicine will function will require *disruptive* changes to the way medicine works. This book presents my view of how these changes could occur without creating a greater burden on physicians and nurses.

These changes will require new computer software systems. Use of computers in medicine has a long history, but this history has all occurred in my lifetime and I have direct experience in the implementation or creation of many of these computer software systems. I have served as a programmer, business analyst, software developer, system implementer, student, patient and patient advocate.

In 1968, Berkeley Scientific Laboratories developed the first on-line clinical laboratory data processing system directly recording information from clinical laboratory instruments. I worked on this system.

In the 70's, the US Air Force Military Airlift Command (MAC) was one of the first, if not the first, to attempt to create an enterprise-wide software system for the entire organization. They created a high-level, but detailed, document, called a *requirements document,* describing how the software system would function in all areas of its organization. I worked in development of this document.

At an Air Force think tank, I developed new ideas for networking computers. At that time, I attended the very first public presentation of Arpanet, a military network of computers that formed the basis for the current Internet.

In 1981, I wrote a successful proposal for an automated patient medical record for King Faisal Hospital in Riyadh, Saudi Arabia. We considered both the Technicon system and an IBM system at that time, choosing the latter.

In 1982, I began working at Kaiser Permanente, Northern California as a business analyst and software developer in the development of an enterprise-wide (multiple facility) appointment system which optimizes physician schedules and results in an enterprise-wide physician time card. The databases I helped design incorporated Kaiser business rules describing how Kaiser functions and were the basis for all later Kaiser Northern California clinic databases. As part of these efforts, I interviewed many nurses and physicians.

I married a paraplegic who developed a number of major health problems. I was a patient advocate for her and a patient myself.

I have taken over a hundred college-level medically related courses from the University of California at San Francisco's Mini Med School, from University of California Extension and from the Great Courses video courses. These courses have ranged from epidemiology and wilderness medicine to immunology and molecular biology to grand rounds and psychiatric and cancer treatments.

In 2000, I worked on automation of Kaiser's medical records, including doing a study to describe in detail how all Kaiser ancillary service software systems—including its hospital, clinical laboratory, pharmacy, and anatomic pathology systems—would interface with such an automated medical record system.

I wrote a book (McGuire, 2015) which presents a requirements document for changes to medicine similar to those described in this book. The present book describes many of these changes in a more understandable way.

This book is dedicated to Bonnie Chin McGuire, my deceased wife.

Note that medical examples are used to illustrate general concepts presented in this book. Medically related information in the examples should not be used to prevent, prognose, diagnose or treat any disease.

ENVISIONING MEDICINE IN THE FUTURE

# 1. Problems with Current Medicine

The following are problems with current medicine (McGuire, 2015) for which this book proposes solutions, followed by names I give to these solutions:

1. No complete patient medical record (*Universal Patient Medical Record*)
2. Lack of direct communication of orders and return of results with commercial ancillary service organizations
3. A patient's significant health problems and descriptions of them are inadequate (*significant health problems*, a *longitudinal disease history* for each)
4. Limited support for extended care occurring beyond a short period of time (*case* and *episode of care*)
5. No support for physicians working together in the care of a patient (*virtual organization*)
6. No support for care when a patient changes medical organizations (*case* and *episode of care*)
7. No support for care occurring in multiple medical organizations (*center of medical expertise, virtual organization*)
8. Inadequate support for *clinical checking* of medications during ordering of medications (e.g., checking for drug interactions or drug allergies). Inadequate checking for duplicate medications or other orders (order checking using information in the *Universal Patient Medical Record*)
9. Inadequate periodic review of an individual's medications, especially those having a lot of medications (*consulting pharmacists*)
10. Ignoring quality of life when measuring quality of care, only using mortality (longevity) (*quality-of-life* measures)
11. Care at the end of life needs to be improved.

12. Emphasis on treating the sick with little emphasis on keeping individuals well.

13. Lack of medical information at the cellular—as opposed to the tissue-level, such as the patient's genome (*biomarkers* in the *Universal Patient Medical Record*)

14. Communication with relatives that they may share a gene variant that could cause disease is lacking.

15. Little current support for treating diseases that do not have obvious symptoms yet but can be predicted and treated (e.g., colon cancer can be treated through colonoscopies by removing polyps that may later turn into cancer (*early treatment diseases*)

16. Lack of approaches to optimize physician time (*physician schedules*)

17. No complete research database

18. No ability to identify best care practices based upon care given to previous patients

19. Little ability to evaluate physicians to determine if they are providing good patient care and inconsistent recording of outcomes which makes doing so difficult to do

20. Patient care in rural areas is often poor, and physicians in rural areas may suffer from lack of advancement.

21. There is less than ideal interaction between medicine and public health.

22. Physicians do not spend enough time identifying confirmed diagnoses in place of differential diagnoses, so medical information is not as correct as it could be.

23. There is no ability for a patient to see his/her complete medical record or do research.

24. There is no way for a patient to have wrong medical information audited and corrected (*physician health advisor / auditor*).

25. No approach to handling complicated medical problems.

26. *Artificial intelligence (AI)* in medicine are programs that assist physicians in making diagnostic and treatment decisions. There are concerns about such programs including that AI is often a "black box."

# ENVISIONING MEDICINE IN THE FUTURE

27.

# 2. The Need for a Complete Patient Medical Record

Today, most medical organizations have gotten away from paper medical records and use computerized electronic medical record systems (EMRs). The U.S. government has encouraged the use of such systems, no matter how large or small these systems are.

If an individual is seen as a patient in different medical organizations, s/he is unlikely to have a complete medical record available at either medical organization. Today EMRs often take care of this problem by allowing the EMR system where the patient is currently being seen to get medical information from the EMR system of the medical organization where the patient is routinely seen for care. This concept is called *interoperability*.

There are a number of problems with interoperability:

- Instead of one pile of basically unreadable medical records, you have multiple piles.

- There is unlikely to be a complete summary of important medical information, such as current medications, past visits, preventive care, allergies, etc., that can be trusted, even if there is such a summary for the medical organization where the patient is normally seen.

- There may be limited ability to have interoperability for smaller-scale EMR systems.

- There are security concerns with such transfers.

I propose that there be a centrally located *Universal Patient Medical Record (UPMR)* for each patient, outside all EMR systems in a *secure healthcare network*. Each UPMR for a patient would be built from physician and other inputs into EMR systems, with UPMR information for a patient being available to each physician caring for the patient. The centrally located UPMR through the network would only be directly available to users of EMR systems, not users outside an EMR.

The UPMR for a patient would provide a comprehensive summary of patient medical information and through this summary would provide the ability of a physician to retrieve medical records (source documents) from EMR systems at other medical organizations. I call this summary a *clinical summary*.

A connection between an EMR and the centrally located UPMR would not be over the Internet but instead by a point-to-point connection. A *point-to-point connection* (Finch, 2023) is "a private data connection between two locations that does not cross the public Internet."

Again, UPMR information for a patient would only be available to an EMR user caring for the patient by point-to-point communication through an EMR system, and thus would not be directly available through an EMR to anyone using the Internet.

# 3. Electronic Medical Record Systems (EMRs)

For there to be a complete UPMR for a patient built from EMR inputs every medical organization must use an EMR system.

Today, many large medical organizations use large-scale EMR systems, Epic and Cerner, with these systems connected to ancillary clinical systems to do ordering and return of results (e.g., clinical lab tests, X-rays or MRIs, prescriptions) and to handle hospital admissions. Other medical organizations either have smaller scale EMR systems or none at all.

To minimize the number of point-to-point connections between EMR systems and the UPMR—and minimize security concerns with such interfaces—I propose that smaller-scale medical organizations use shared EMR systems handling EMR services for many medical organizations. I call an EMR system for one medical organization, a *dedicated EMR system*, and an EMR system for multiple different medical organizations, a *utility EMR system*.

A utility EMR could also handle administrative functions for a medical organization such as billing, insurance payments, and payment to the medical organization.

To minimize the possibility that an unauthorized person could get access to the UPMR information for a patient through a remote EMR system, reading it or updating it, I propose the following:

An individual, together with a medical organization, would identify medical organizations where the individual is normally seen for care. At these medical organizations, the EMR would be able to view the UPMR. When a patient is seen by a physician at another medical organization, the patient must provide biometric information (e.g., facial, voice, iris, palm vein patterns) before the physician has access to the patient's UPMR.

A physician receiving an outside referral from a physician who is authorized to see the UPMR will also be able to see the UPMR so they may respond to the referral.

# 4. Medical Records Within EMRs (Source Documents)

Most patient medical information today is in the form of encounter- and consult-oriented documents that I call *source documents*. Source documents (currently referred to as "medical records") will continue to exist in the future and will be kept by each medical organization.

*Source documents* that currently exist in most completely automated EMR systems today will continue to exist in this proposal, and consist of the following types of documents:

- Medical record forms with medical information entered through an EMR system: in PDF or other textual format with identification of data fields that can support retrieval (e.g., retrieval by encounter identifier).

- Diagnostic digital images (e.g., X-rays, MRIs): in DICOM format, where *DICOM (Digital Imaging and Communications in Medicine)* is a recognized digital standard for digitized diagnostic images (Pianykh,2012).

- Scanned medical records: usually in TIFF format with inclusion of extracted data that is important information, especially information to be used as key data to enable storage and future retrieval (e.g., identification of the patient and the encounter). This is written information from the patient or other information not entered through the EMR system.

Often source documents are in the format of a SOAP note (Podder et al., 2023), where SOAP stands for the four parts of the document:

1. **Subjective:** information contributed by the patient, from the patient's point of view.

2. **Objective:** data acquired by inspection, percussion, auscultation and palpation and from laboratory, radiology and other diagnostic

tests. (Auscultation is listening to sounds from the heart, lungs, or other organs, typically with a stethoscope.)

3. **Assessment**: assessment of the problem that is an analysis of the subjective and objective data.
4. **Plan:** a care plan for the encounter, which may recommend further diagnostic work, therapy, and education or counseling.

As is true today, source documents in 2030 will be legal documents identifying what happened during the encounter and cannot be changed once signed off by the physician. Corrections to a source document that has been signed off must be made via an addendum source document.

# 5. A Clinical Summary

The principal part of the UPMR would be a *clinical summary,* a summary of patient medical information.

Today, when two EMR systems transport medical information from one EMR to the other, the information transferred is likely a set of encounters- and consult-based medical records (i.e., *source documents*). In such a case, after the transfer there is no summary of a patient's medical information such as a list of medications taken, allergies, and health problems.

If the EMR system also created summary information in the system it transferred information to, there is no guarantee that there is not additional patient medical information in other EMR systems, so the summary is not guaranteed to be complete.

In the future, all EMR systems will interface with the secure healthcare network providing summary information from all medical organizations where the patient received care. There will be, along with other patient medical information in the secure healthcare network, a *clinical summary* that identifies all the patient's significant health problems and may identify other health problems; physicians who regularly provide care for the patient including contact information; a complete list of the patient's medications; test results; next due and completed dates for preventive health interventions; allergies; recent orders; outside referrals; and a complete list of a patient's encounters with health personnel (outpatient visits and hospital stays) identifying where the patient was seen for care and identifying the healthcare practitioner and nature of the visit.

The clinical summary would include identifier information (UPMR identifier, identifiers at each of the medical organizations), and standard descriptors such as birthdate and gender.)

The *clinical summary* would be available to any physician and other authorized medical professional providing care for the patient.

The *clinical summary* will be available during a patient encounter. An *encounter* is a meeting of an individual with medical personnel whether this is face-to-face or via telehealth or a communication between a patient and medical personnel. There are three types of encounters:

- An *outpatient visit*—an emergency department or telehealth visit is also considered an outpatient visit.
- An *inpatient stay*—a stay in the hospital or the new concept of "hospital at home" (which will be discussed later in this book).
- A communication—an email, telephone advice nurse communication recording or other communication between a patient and medical personnel.

In addition to being available to physicians in contact with the patient, the *clinical summary* will also be available to a physician receiving a *referral* from a physician who has seen the patient. A *referral* is either a request that the referred-to physician provide consultation advice to the referring physician or that the referred-to physician set up a meeting with the patient. The clinical summary will be available for the referred-to physician to process the referral. Interspersed with the encounters in the clinical summary will be *consults,* where a *consult* is a consultation response back to the referring physician from the referred-to physician as a result of a consultation request.

The clinical summary will include three levels of health problems: (1) significant health problems: (2) less significant health problems: and (3) other categories defined by physicians. For each health problem there will be a list of all encounters and consults where care or advice was provided for the patient for the health problem.

When a patient receives care for the very first time, information will be collected to initiate the clinical summary and biometric information to identify the patient.

An individual can identify a medical organization as a *home medical organization* where the individual is normally seen for care. An individual who no longer goes to this medical organization may have it removed as a home medical organization. Ideally, at the time an individual identifies a home medical organization, the individual should be assigned to a primary care physician to oversee the individual's care at that medical organization.

The clinical summary will be available for view by authorized physicians at the individual's home facilities. The clinical summary will also be available to a physician at a non-home facility when the patient is physically seen for care, and the clinical summary will be available for a limited time when a non-home facility physician receives a referral to allow the physician to process the referral. This approach prevents fraudulent access to a patient's medical information from other EMR systems.

EMR systems will still function as they did in the past, producing medical records for each patient encounter or consult, and saving these medical records within the EMR system. An authorized medical professional viewing a clinical summary could select an encounter or consult listed in the clinical summary and retrieve and display the medical records for the selected encounter or consult. Again, I call such encounter- and consult-oriented medical records *source documents*. It is expected that most of the time, the clinical summary will provide sufficient information for patient care without retrieval and display of source documents.

# 6. Proposed New Infrastructure for Sharing Patient Medical Information

It is proposed that in the future there will only be large size EMR systems. Most large medical organizations will have their own EMR systems; other medical organizations will share EMR system services. A medical organization-owned EMR system is a *dedicated EMR system,* and the shared one is a *utility EMR system.*

A government-provided and supported healthcare network, that I call a *secure healthcare network*, will connect with these EMR systems, enabling the controlled display of a patient's combined medical information gathered from all medical organizations where the patient received care.

The network will collect medical information on each patient from the EMR systems after medical personnel caring for the patient enter the information through the EMR system and sign it off as complete and correct. From this patient's medical information, collected from all medical organizations, the healthcare network will develop a *clinical summary in the UPMR* that will summarize medical information for the patient. The UPMR could also contain additional information and provide additional services.

Information in the secure healthcare network will not be on the Internet and will only be available to vetted EMR systems. Limiting EMR systems to major large-scale brand systems that have been vigorously vetted for security threats and keeping the secure healthcare network separate from the Internet will limit unauthorized access by hackers both to information in the EMR systems and in the healthcare network.

A patient's *home medical organization* is a medical organization where the patient is normally seen for care.

To protect secure healthcare information from hackers who have availability to an EMR system, a patient's medical information on the secure network will only be available to (1) authorized medical personnel at the patient's *home medical organization*; (2) authorized medical personnel at a non-home medical organization when the patient physically shows up for care; or (3) a physician on a limited basis who receives an authorized referral. When a patient shows up for care at a *remote medical organization*, the patient must provide *biometric information* for the EMR system for the patient's medical information in the secure healthcare network to be seen. *Biometrics* is an automated way of recognizing a person by physical information such as the person's face, iris, fingerprints, handwriting or voice.

Patient medical information in the network will be mirrored in an EMR system for a patient's home medical organization, producing a mirrored UPMR database for that medical organization. The network would send down any updates as they occur; the secure healthcare network would send down any changes to the UPMR, and any source documents created at a medical organization that is not the patient's home medical organization and add it to home medical organization UPMR information. The mirrored database is meant for exclusive use of that medical organization but can only be modified by the secure healthcare network.

Today medical organizations do display medical record information to patients over the Internet using medical organization security measures. A medical organization can choose to include information from the patient's mirrored UPMR.

A dedicated EMR system enables the EMR system to directly connect to the medical organization's pharmacy, clinical laboratory and other ancillary system software systems, enabling ancillary system ordering and return of results within the organization.

# 7. An Overview of Other Envisioned Future Changes

Besides a UPMR, which includes a Clinical Summary, this book envisions other changes in medicine in the future, some which could be included in the UPMR and others which could occur without there being a UPMR.

## *Commercial Ancillary Service Ordering*

Unlike medical organization ancillary care systems directly connected to an EMR, it is proposed that commercial ancillary care systems receive orders from EMR systems through the secure healthcare network and return results through the secure healthcare network. This would minimize the number of connections to commercial ancillary care systems, as otherwise there would be required to be connections to multiple EMR systems.

The UPMR having a complete list of medications and recent orders would enable checking for medication problems (e.g., drug interactions) and duplicate orders.

## *Significant Health Problems for a Patient*

Today in an EMR system a list of a patient's health problems may be incomplete or not exist. A complete list of a patient's significant health problems will be kept in the UPMR with a disease history for each built by physicians over time. Currently disease histories are encounter-based and occur in each SOAP note created during an encounter.

A disease history in a SOAP note changes every encounter. A disease history in the UPMR is ongoing. To distinguish the disease history in the UPMR in this book it will be called *a longitudinal disease history*, but often just *disease history*.

## Extended Care and Increased Physician Responsibility for Care

Medicine today is single encounter-oriented, with the patient medical record structured to support one encounter at a time. The problem with this single encounter orientation is that it often takes a number of encounters to get a correct diagnosis or that care for a medical condition could extend over many encounters before the medical situation can be resolved. Further, for chronic conditions, care for the condition is needed over an extended period of time, even over the patient's lifetime. In the future, physicians should take more responsibility in providing long-term care for the patient.

The book *From Chaos to Care* by David Lawrence (Lawrence, 2003), the former head of Kaiser Permanente, describes good care for a patient with a particular medical problem: care that is described by consistency (the care is consistent until it is deliberately changed), continuity (the patient is not forgotten), and coordination (there is someone to coordinate the care). I call these the three C's. In this book I propose two data structures in the UPMR to support such care for a patient's medical concern or problem, a *case* and *episode of care*.

These data structures would identify the patient and medical concern or problem; the physician coordinating care (for coordination); contact information for the coordinator; a care plan for all physicians dealing with this problem to follow except for emerging situations (for consistency); a list of related encounters; the next encounter (for continuity) and an optional list of team members. An *episode of care* would be for a problem that is expected to be resolved (e.g., a wrist fracture) while a *case* would be for a chronic or long-lasting condition.

Note that a care plan in a SOAP note—like a disease history—is for a single encounter, while a care plan in a case or episode of care is good until it is changed by the coordinating physician.

## Physicians Working Together in Care

Physicians often work together in a hierarchy, sort of like supervisor and employee but only for a specific patient. For example, for a patient in the hospital, an attending physician most often recruits physicians of various specialties to resolve a patient's medical problem(s). The attending physician functions as a supervisor of these physicians. I propose a data structure called a *virtual organization* that identifies this hierarchy, with the supervising physician being told of any time a supervised physician makes changes to the patient's medical records and vice versa. Associated with any physician in a virtual organization could be a case or episode of care.

## Care Across Medical Organizations

Cases, episodes of care, and virtual organizations could either be in the EMR system to support care within a single medical organization or in the UPMR to support care in multiple medical organizations.

## Transferring Care Between Medical Organizations

The book *Mistreated* by Dr. Robert Pearl (Pearl, 2017) describes how care can go wrong when a patient moves to a different medical organization, which may benefit from a case or episode of care being in the UPMR. I propose that when a patient moves to a new medical organization that a new coordinator be established for the case or episode of care in the new medical organization, with the new coordinator contacting the previous one and continuing use of the case or episode of care in the new medical organization.

## Order Checking

No EMR system is guaranteed to have a complete list of medications, allergies, and current orders for a patient; the UPMR does. This book thus proposes that orders, including medication orders, be checked by the secure healthcare network before being made. Duplicate orders could be detected, and with a complete list of medications and allergies, drug interactions and drug allergies could be detected. Order checking would apply to both orders with commercial and local ancillary care systems.

## Overall Management of a Patient's Medications

This book proposes new types of physicians and medical workers, including a pharmacist consultant. A *pharmacist consultant* will meet periodically with each patient receiving many medications to determine medications that are not needed, are needed, cause problems, or can be replaced with more effective ones, with a report back to the patient's primary care physician to make changes in the medications.

## Quality-of-Life Used in Care Evaluation

Besides morbidity and mortality (longevity) quality-of-life will be used more often in evaluating medical care.

## Improved End-of-Life Decisions

Quality of life at the end of life will be more of a consideration in the future than today when the current emphasis is on longevity.

## Keeping Patients Well

Although a patient is often given written information on how to treat a current sickness, patients are not often given other information on how to keep well.

## Genetics and the Genome and Other Biomarkers

The UPMR will include overall biomarkers for an individual, biomarkers that are fixed and do not change. Overall biomarkers are used for patient care and research (e.g., birthdate, gender, and perhaps genome.)

Should a patient's genome be part of the UPMR? If so, genetic variants that are associated with disease can be identified. For example, gene variants sometimes cause a disease (cystic fibrosis, Down syndrome, hemophilia, Huntington's disease, ALS, Williams syndrome); variants such as BRCA1 and BRCA2 predispose a person to breast cancer; and gene variants can predict the effects of dosages of active and prodrugs.

## *Relatives Sharing Genetic Information*

Presented is an approach to sharing genetic information among relatives that gets around some possible problems; including that a patient may not want to share genetic information or a relative not wanting to know the information.

## *Early Treatment*

Today, colon cancer can be treated before it occurs. During a colonoscopy, polyps (abnormal growths) that could later turn into colon cancer can be detected and removed.

In the future it may be possible to predict and treat more diseases before symptoms become obvious or before they occur. This book identifies how to do so and problems that could occur in doing so. I call these early treatment diseases.

## *Optimizing Physician Time*

Optimizing physician time will lower healthcare costs and minimize any shortage of physicians.

The author has been involved in the creation of a physician appointment scheduling system that optimized physician time without overburdening the physicians, which saved a medical organization a lot of money. The approach did not depend upon a UPMR. This system is described in detail later in this book.

*Artificial* intelligence (AI) programs are computer programs that will assist physicians in making diagnostic and treatment decisions. AI will free physician time.

## Researching Best Care and Prognoses

A physician can refer a patient to a *physician consultant* and a *physician analyst* to use the patient's mirrored UPMR database to select similar patients with the same medical problem from a de-identified research database created from UPMRs to evaluate best care for the patient for the medical problem or to generate a prognosis for the patient's medical problem. *De-identified* means all information identifying patients has been removed (McCallister, 2010).

## Accountability

According to the book *Unaccountable* (Makary, 2013), there are some physicians who perform poorly on procedures without this being recognized by patients. This book discusses evaluation of physicians in the performance of procedures based upon data in a medical organization's source documents (to find a procedure performed by a particular physician) and by longitudinal disease histories (to identify ultimate outcomes of the procedures.)

## Patient Care in Rural Areas

Patient care is often lacking in rural areas with few clinics, few physicians and even fewer specialists. Advancement as a physician may be difficult in a rural area. This book proposes ways to revolutionize rural medical care.

## Public Health

Medicine can be changed to provide more information to public health and public health can be changed in response to help physicians recognize patients who live in areas where a particular disease is prevalent.

## *Confirmed Diagnoses*

Because there are many similar diseases that can be treated the same way and because there may be a number of tentative or differential diagnoses, then in source documents there is often no one confirmed diagnosis but many differential and tentative ones. Medical research may then suffer from the lack of a confirmed diagnosis. This book presents ways to increase the chance of a clear confirmed diagnosis.

## *Patient Ability to See and Audit the UPMR*

Today, many medical organizations allow a patient to see his/her medical information over the Internet using security measures controlled by the medical organization. The patient's mirrored UPMR database is another database owned by the patient's home medical organization; that medical organization could choose to include this information in a display to the patient, enabling the patient to audit and a physician to update the patient's UPMR.

A *physician health advisor/auditor* is a physician who meets with patients on how to keep well and enables patient review of their medical information in their mirrored UPMR database either at the patient's home medical organization or at an EPR utility organization. Suggestions on corrections to information in the UPMR could be made, sending these suggestions to the individual's primary care physician.

## *Handling Complicated Medical Problems*

When a patient comes in with an unusual disease, presents with different symptoms than normal, or has a different disease than originally expected, then the physician must go beyond giving care based upon care for similar patients and do an analysis.

This analysis could be done with the assistance of a *physician consultant* and *physician analyst* doing research.

## Increased Use of Artificial Intelligence

*Artificial intelligence (AI)* programs in medicine are computer programs that make diagnostic and treatment recommendations (Ahuja,2019), whereas such decisions were previously all done by physicians. AI can also assist physicians in entering medical record documentation such as SOAP notes and hospital discharge summaries.

An example of artificial intelligence is analysis of radiological images (mammograms) for breast cancer based upon the program learning from past images and associated outcomes. (Ahuja, 2019) An AI program can search medical literature or patient medical data bases and present diagnostic or care recommendations in educated prose.

Besides being used by medical organizations, AI programs can also be used directly by an individual. For example, an Apple watch can identify atrial fibrillation in a wearer, which can indicate that the individual has a greater risk of stroke than other individuals (Pepplinkhuize et al., 2022).

Many new data centers are being built for AI because many AI systems perform "massive concurrent searches for information" (Montie, 2023). Since the secure healthcare network itself requires many concurrent processes for many patients, the network could potentially be piggybacked off these data centers

AI programs will be used more in the future because they can free expensive physician time, saving medical organizations money.

# 8. Commercial Ancillary Services and Order Checking

An EMR system could send orders to commercial ancillary service systems through the secure healthcare network and receive back results through the secure healthcare network. This would minimize the number of connections to ancillary care systems and more seamlessly allow the secure healthcare network to do clinical and order checking.

As examples of ordering and return of results, clinical lab tests, x-rays or MRIs could be ordered, and results of these tests could be returned. For a prescription (medication order), the results would be that the medication was picked up.

(Ordering and return of results for non-commercial ancillary service systems that are run by the medical organization may have direct connections with the medical organization's EMR system to handle ordering and return of results. A medical organization ancillary service system can optionally be treated like a commercial system, with ordering and return of result through the secure healthcare network.)

All orders, commercial or otherwise, directly handled by the secure healthcare network, will be checked by the network. Physicians at two different medical organizations may issue the same medical order for a patient (e.g., prescribe the same medication or order the same blood test within a given time frame). Because only the secure healthcare network, through the patient's UPMR, will be able to detect such a duplicate order within two different medical organizations, the secure healthcare network will be responsible for reporting a duplicate order to the ordering physician.

The secure healthcare network accumulates a complete list of the medications for a patient by combining the medications ordered at each medical organization where the patient was seen. The secure healthcare network will have a complete list of a patient's medications, while an EMR system may not. The secure healthcare network will thus be given the responsibility of checking for medication interactions as part of prescription ordering.

The secure healthcare network will likewise check for drug allergies, as unlike the network, any EMR system may not have a complete list of reported drug allergies.

The secure healthcare network could inform a physician when a patient fails to pick up or continue a vital medication (e.g., eye drops to halt the progression of glaucoma.)

For a prescription, a physician may give the number of refills and minimum time between refills. Before issuing a medication, a commercial pharmacy will ask the secure healthcare network if there are any more refills, and if so, the earliest date for the next refill. The pharmacist in consultation with the patient may call up the ordering physician to resolve any problems.

It is feasible that a commercial ancillary services organization (e.g., Walgreens or CVS) could have a single connection or only a few connections to the secure healthcare network, yet support ordering and results returns from many different locations.

# 9. Physicians as Story Tellers: Significant Health Problems and Disease Histories

In the UPMR would be a list of significant health problems for a patient together with other health problems, some of which could turn into significant health problems. It is anticipated that the possible health problems will be standardized with the ability to add new ones in the future.

For each health problem there could be a longitudinal disease history of the problem, telling a story of the problem over many encounters, unlike a source document that is a legal document that tells what happened during a single encounter where a source document is signed off at the end of an encounter so it can no longer be changed. A longitudinal disease history's sole purpose is to support patient care. It may be updated if necessary to ensure the disease history is correct; for example, it would be changed when a confirmed diagnosis was found to replace a differential diagnosis.

Many diseases last over a significant period before their true nature is determined. Today, with care being given at the single encounter level, the story of the disease is often lost, or parts of the story are lost, hindering better care that can be given with a more complete and accurate disease history that records the history over multiple encounters.

Currently, disease histories in source documents come mostly from the patient. There are two problems with this: (1) people, in this case patients, don't always have good memories, and (2) patients often don't know a lot about medicine. Further, disease history information collected during an encounter is often only what's necessary for the encounter.

Consider a woman who is a paraplegic with information collected under the category "paraplegia." She became a paraplegic at thirty; she had an operation to stabilize her back; she learned to sit up in bed; she learned how to use a wheelchair and care for herself; she had urinary tract infections; she developed pressure ulcers; she developed sepsis from a deep infected pressure ulcer; she recovered from sepsis; she broke bones due to falls; she developed blood clots; etc. Stories of other paraplegics could be compared and used by a physician to inform a patient who just became a paraplegic on how to avoid these problems a paraplegic could face later in life.

The paraplegic woman had another healthcare story under the category "heart problem." She had mitral valve regurgitation; she has been short of breath; she had pulmonary edema while on a ventilator for the sepsis caused by the pressure ulcer; she had a heart attack followed by a pulmonary embolism (blood clot in her lung); she fell and had an open wound followed by a second bout of sepsis. The last fall was related to the heart problem, in that it caused her to be so weak that she could no longer be lifted by her caregiver.

It was unclear if the pulmonary edema (water in the lungs) was due to the heart problem, too much IV fluid for fighting the bout of sepsis or both; thus, the "sepsis caused by the pressure ulcer" was part of both stories.

I have a healthcare story under the category "knee fracture." I was involved in a motorbike accident when I was 20; my knee was shattered; I had an operation to fix the fracture; I limped for a year; after 2 years, I was able to play basketball; I developed arthritis; I eventually had a hard time running; I then had a hard time walking for a distance; I developed sciatica in my other leg; I took an opioid medication for pain; I had a knee replacement; etc. (My knee replacement could have been unsuccessful, in which case there would be another *event*: a follow-up operation would likely have been done to re-do the knee replacement.)

Comparing the stories of others with such a knee fracture could enable a physician to tell a patient who has such a knee injury, a probable future course of his problem.

A son brought in his elderly father for care, as his father was having memory problems. The first physician diagnosed the father as having Alzheimer's disease. The second physician tested to see if a medication side effect was responsible for the memory problem. After changing medications, the memory problems improved but did not go away.

The elderly man thus has a healthcare story connected with a memory problem, with Alzheimer's at the last time of diagnosis assumed to be a 50% probability and a transient problem (such as a medication side effect) assumed to be a 50% probability for the problem. This may be an ongoing story, with the future determining if indeed the patient has Alzheimer's. The disease history might initially be put under the category, "potential memory problem," with a possible change to the title as more is known.

When it is known whether a health problem is transient or permanent, the category of the problem might need to be modified when more is known, and the story might need to be changed.

A patient was diagnosed with Lyme disease. Based upon a later interview with the patient, a date on which the tick bite occurred could be estimated based upon when the patient was out in the woods, adding another event in the story.

These are shortened examples of healthcare stories, each associated with a particular milestone medical condition, that could include related associated *events* collected over time, such as the following: (1) the milestone medical condition (e.g., knee injury); (2) a significant medical condition associated with the initial medical condition (e.g., arthritis); (3) a follow-on medical condition to the secondary medical condition; (4) medication taken as a result of a medical condition; (5) a side effect of such a medication; (6) a procedure as a result of a medical condition; (7) a new medical condition resulting from a procedure; (8) a related medically significant life event (e.g., death of a spouse, physical abuse); or (9) a related medically significant lifestyle or change in lifestyle (e.g., smokes tobacco or initiates an exercise or stress management program). When an event is added to a disease history, the encounter in which the event occurred will be automatically recorded.

Added to each of these healthcare stories periodically over time could be 0.0 to 1.0 quality of life outcome measures, values both related to the individual's overall health and to the milestone medical condition or to a subsequent related event.

Additionally, for the milestone medical condition and each subsequent event, associated biomarkers could be recorded (e.g., blood pressure for sepsis).

A biomarker is defined as a "cellular, biochemical, molecular or genetic characteristic or alteration by which a normal, abnormal, or simply biologic process can be recognized, or monitored" (McGuire, 2015).

This information would be collected by physicians bit by bit over the individual's lifetime. For a milestone medical condition, I call this set of information a *longitudinal disease history* for that milestone medical condition and, after this point in this book, I will use the shortened term *disease history*.

Today, *big data* is used for the analysis of patient medical information. *Big data* is a large data set (e.g., all a patient's source documents) that can computationally reveal patterns, trends, and associations. In the future, *longitudinal disease histories* will replace big data in medicine for the selection of a category of patients when doing this analysis, and it will be the primary source of data for analysis rather than source documents.

An important part of a longitudinal disease history are biomarkers taken before or after events in the disease history. For example, an event could be a procedure with related biomarkers recorded both before and after the procedure; with this information perhaps automatically retrieved from source documents.

Medical conditions, procedures, medications and other events will be standardized so they can be recognized by software, during research.

Based upon information entered through the EMR system, the system can question the physician on whether a new significant health problem and disease history should be added. Upon adding a significant health problem, the system can look back to add previously associated events. For example, upon a confirmed diagnosis of breast cancer, the system could include the previous mammogram.

Based upon medical research, a new medical condition that could be a result of an event in a longitudinal disease history will be automatically added to the disease history. As an example: For a disease history for a cataract, a retinal detachment that occurs after a cataract surgery event would be automatically recorded in the disease history, given the retinal detachment could result from the cataract surgery. Conversely, a disease history for a retinal detachment could look back to see if there was cataract surgery and include it in the detached retina disease history.

The system at any time could suggest that the physician collect specific biomarker information from the patient to be included in the disease history.

These processes can be collectively viewed as *connecting the dots*: "looking for events and connections between events in longitudinal disease histories and including biomarkers."

Big data is used in medicine for "predictive modeling and clinical decision support, disease or safety surveillance, public health, and research" (Belle et al., 2015). In the future, this information will be developed from disease histories.

Disease histories will be correctable and will be used to assist in patient care rather than being legal documents. The source documents will remain as the legal documents that identify what occurred during an encounter. Advantages of disease histories over big data (the collective source documents) are that disease histories distinguish differential diagnoses from confirmed diagnoses and disease histories can be corrected for errors, which is not true for big data.

Each of the healthcare stories can be changed as more is known. For example, if the elderly man with a memory problem was confirmed to have Alzheimer's disease, then the title of the story, the disease history, might be changed from "potential memory problem" to "Alzheimer's disease."

When a physician is reviewing a disease history, the physician can select an event to see the source documents for the encounter in which the event was reported.

A *physician health advisor/auditor* will meet periodically with individuals, having access to information in the patient's mirrored UPMR. Together with the patient he/she can suggest new significant health problems and/or new longitudinal disease histories. He/she can recommend updates to the individual's stories in disease histories, making each story more accurate, comprehensible and comprehensive. This information would be sent to the patient's personal physician for possible additions or changes to the UPMR.

How could well-developed disease histories be used?

Later in this book I will demonstrate how disease histories could be used to improve and evaluate patient care. For now, I contend that they can be used in the following ways:

- A complete, accurate history of a disease: Disease histories can be used to provide a complete and accurate history of a patient's disease, supporting patient care.

- Prognosis: Combining disease histories of similar patients with the same disease can produce a prognosis for a patient.

- Intervention evaluation: Two interventions for the same disease and category of patients can be evaluated by using disease histories of these patients.

- Accountability: By identifying the physicians performing or recommending procedures or other interventions in disease histories, a physician's possible competence can be evaluated based upon the outcomes.

- Prevention: By identifying future medical conditions related to a medical problem and devising countermeasures to avoid these medical conditions. Using this information on countermeasures, a physician can advise a patient with the medical problem on how to avoid these related medical conditions that could occur in the future.

Some of the above require gathering information from disease histories of other patients. In order to do this the identities of these patients must not be available during the analysis. One approach is to develop a research data base that includes disease histories but excludes the identities of the patients. HIPAA provides a way to do this.

(HIPAA is the Health Insurance Portability and Accounting Act of 1996.)

HIPAA requires removal of identification information for patients in research databases by a process called *de-identification* when the information is moved to the research database (Institutional Review Board, 2003).

AI programs could potentially produce the longitudinal patient histories in place of physicians. When a physician signs off an encounter identifying the encounter with one or more health problems or identifies a confirmed diagnosis, an AI program could create a new health problem, substitute one health problem with another or automatically add to a disease history associated with the encounter.

**ENVISIONING MEDICINE IN THE FUTURE**

# 10. The Three C's

Today, medical care occurs one encounter at a time. Although medical organizations today do support continuing care for an existing medical problem, they most often do not provide a formal mechanism to ensure that this continuing care occurs. These formal mechanisms to support care across encounters will be available in the future.

A physician may indeed provide care for her patient's medical condition only for one encounter, e.g., a urinary infection. On the other hand, the patient may have a significant health problem that requires care over numerous encounters or even over the patient's lifetime. In such a situation, an encounter-based care plan could be inefficient; instead, it may be better to have a single care plan for the medical condition that lasts across many encounters.

Consider some problems that could occur if such care was given one encounter at a time: (1) If the patient was seen by different physicians, then the care plan might change with every encounter, possibly with one care plan contradicting the other. (2) There would be no physician managing care. (3) The patient might be seen only once or a few times and then forgotten (Lawrence, 2003).

In the future, with *health problems* identified in the *clinical summary*, there could be associated information I call either an *episode of care* or a *case*. Within the *episode of care* or *case* would be the following information:

- Health problem.
- Managing physician for the episode of care or case and previous managers, including contact information.
- Other team members jointly providing care.
- Care plan for the episode of care or case—a care plan that applies until changed, likely applicable for multiple encounters.
- List of encounters and consults related to the health problem.

- Planned future event to guarantee that the patient will be seen in the future (e.g., an appointment, a referral, search parameters for a future appointment, a future message to the manager, a future message to the patient).
- Information on a no-show for a planned appointment.

The difference between an *episode of care* and a *case* is that an episode of care will have a final outcome, most often that the patient is cured or is stable, while a case lasts for a long time, even a lifetime. A *case* is for a chronic health problem.

An *episode of care* or a *case* ensures that the following three things will happen, which I call the *three C's*:

- Coordination of care: There is a physician to manage and coordinate care.
- Continuity of care: The managing physician ensures that the patient comes in for care as necessary; the patient is not forgotten.
- Consistency of care: the care plan is not inconsistently changed every encounter.

The managing physician would be responsible for the care plan for the episode of care or case. The care plan may change, but often it will remain the same across encounters.

Non-managing physicians would have an obligation, except in emergent situations, to follow the care plan in the episode of care or the case. Such a physician could disagree with the care plan, in which case she could record a second opinion, sending it to the managing physician; the managing physician would then have the option to change the episode of care or case care plan. In any case (whether there is a disagreement with the care plan), any visit dealing with the case or episode of care medical condition would result in the managing physician being immediately informed of the visit.

When a non-managing physician is caring for the patient and has a concern about the patient, the physician can use the contact information to consult with the managing physician, who likely has more familiarity with the patient's health problem.

At any time, a patient could request a second opinion by a non-managing physician, in which case the non-managing physician's opinion will be sent to the managing physician, again possibly resulting in a change of the episode of care or case care plan. The managing physician should periodically encourage the patient to seek a second opinion.

Especially for a case, there will likely be many different managing physicians over time, as a case may occur over the patient's lifetime. Further, the patient may change medical organization locations, and this may require a change in the managing physician. Especially when a health problem becomes quiescent, there may be no managing physician.

Besides a next event, also what could be included are "important date(s)." For example, a person with a pacemaker could be checked out periodically. An important date might be the date the battery in the pacemaker should be checked to be replaced, which may only sometimes be the date of the next event.

The patient should be aware that s/he has a case or episode of care. The patient can request a change of physician managers at any time.

Source documents within EMR systems would remain the same as they are today. There would be care plans for encounters in encounter-based (SOAP) source documents in addition to care plans within episodes of care and cases. Like the list of encounters in a clinical summary, an encounter in a case or episode of care list of encounters can be selected by a physician to see all source documents for the encounter.

There will be an additional type of case document for a high utilizer of medical care, especially an individual who makes frequent use of the emergency department, which is often the costliest type of medical care. Some indigent high utilizers together could cost a county millions of dollars in a year (Knight, 2022).

Such *high utilizers* will be assigned a clinical social worker as a case manager and the case will not be for a specific health problem but for all the individual's health problems. The social worker will (1) attempt to get the individual in for care outside the emergency department before a medical condition becomes more acute, saving on the cost of care; (2) seek support such as shelter, food, education or drug counseling to enable the individual to have a healthier life; and (3) guide the individual in lifestyle changes that could avoid medical problems.

Such a case structure for a high utilizer I call an *overall case* and it would be the same as the case structure for a health problem but would not include the health problem, would have the clinical social worker as the manager rather than a physician, and would enable recording of useful information about the patient in place of the case care plan. The clinical social worker would be immediately informed when the individual seeks care at any emergency department and likely would later plan follow-on care to avoid future medical emergencies.

For all patients, continuity of care is a particular problem when a patient changes medical organizations (Pearl, 2017). To ensure continuity of care when there is a change of medical organizations, then a primary care physician at the new organization should consider changing managers for cases and episodes of care with the new managers being at the new medical organization. This should be done in conjunction with the patient, potential new managers and possibly previous managers. Newly assigned physician managers could contact previous managers in the other medical organization to get more information on the patient's care.

One type of planned future event to guarantee that the patient is seen in the future is search parameters for a future appointment. Physician appointment schedules are put out periodically, say every couple of months, so an appointment may not be able to be made for a distant time (e.g., a year from now). What could be done is to save search parameters to search for an appointment at a future date that are initiated when the corresponding physician schedules are released for appointment booking. An appointment is made and the patient is informed of the appointment through mail, email or text. I call the search parameters that are saved a *futures list entry* saved with other futures list entries on a *futures list*.

MICHAEL R. MCGUIRE

# 11. Virtual Organizations

In almost all organizations, an employee has a supervisor who is responsible for guiding the employee in doing his/her job. This requires good communication between the two.

Currently in medicine, especially during stays in the hospital, there is a similar relationship between physicians: the attending physician recruits the needed specialist physicians to provide care for the patient and supervises their care of the patient. The difference between such a relationship and relationships in other organizations is that this relationship is just for the patient and the relationship is a less permanent one.

I call such a relationship, a *virtual organization*. In the future, greater support will be provided for virtual organizations.

Although a virtual organization is less permanent than an employee/supervisor relationship, it could be of much more consequence, as it could negatively affect a person's health. It could even result in mortality if there is not the proper communication between the supervising physician and the other physicians, or if the supervising physician has not recruited the right physicians.

An example of a virtual organization that previously existed was for a recoverable bout of sepsis for my now deceased paraplegic wife. She was confined to bed for a while, and without her knowing it, developed a pressure ulcer that spread down to her hip resulting in the infection of the hip bone and thus the sepsis.

Pressure ulcers (also called pressure sores and bedsores) are "injuries to skin and underlying tissue resulting from prolonged pressure on the skin" (Mayo Clinic, 2023).

Upon entering the hospital, the attending physician recruited an orthopedic surgeon to remove the infection from her hip bone and an osteomyelitis infection specialist to determine the antibiotics to be given to her. See

Figure 1. (In the figure, I included a cardiologist, a specialist I later determined that the patient should have had).

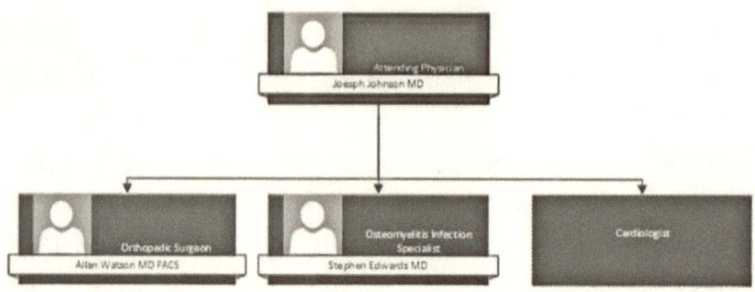

**Figure 1. Virtual Organization Example (Physician Names are Fictitious)**

My wife was put on a ventilator in the ICU and given the antibiotics together with a large amount of fluid to raise her blood pressure. After a while, the attending physician diagnosed her with congestive heart failure due to water in her lungs.

I asked the attending physician why he did not assign a cardiologist. The attending physician said he did not think this was necessary.

My wife indicated she wanted to be off the ventilator, and a nurse called me up saying "your wife wants to die"—I rightly said she just wants to get off the ventilator.

My wife was taken off the ventilator and transferred to a regular hospital bed, putting her into hospice care because they wrongly assumed she wanted to die rather than just being taken off the ventilator. I noticed that she was no longer being given antibiotics. At the same time, the osteomyelitis infection physician came in to visit. He was not told my wife was taken off antibiotics and restarted them again, possibly saving her life. My wife also had a hard time breathing and could only whisper. According to the attending physician, this was due to the congestive heart failure. The osteomyelitis specialist said that the department next door drains fluid from a person's lungs.

My wife was taken temporarily to the department next door where they removed a tremendous amount of fluid from her lungs. Thereafter, she had no trouble breathing or speaking. I had read a medical journal article which said that often, when a patient has severe sepsis, because of the large amount of fluid given to raise the patient's blood pressure, the patient develops fluid in the lungs independent of a heart problem (Kelm et al., 2015). Apparently, this was the case. Perhaps if a cardiologist was assigned, she/he would have recognized this problem. The journal article also stated that this situation of too much fluid in the lungs could cause a patient's death, even when it is not due to a heart problem (Kelm et al., 2015).

So, because the attending physician did not communicate with the osteomyelitis physician about my wife being taken off antibiotics, she could have died. Because the attending physician did not recruit a cardiologist even though he diagnosed her with congestive heart failure, my wife probably unnecessarily suffered from having a hard time breathing and speaking, and there was the chance she might have died due to the excess fluid in her lungs.

Communication between the supervising physician and other physicians, in any case, is essential for good patient care, but providing an automated capability connected with a virtual organization could help in this communication: the supervising physician could be told of any medical records created for the patient by a supervised physician and vice versa, and *messaging* between physicians could be supported.

For each physician in a virtual organization structure, an associated *episode of care* could be identified.

For self-protection, patients and family members should be aware of virtual organizations and support this communication between physicians by communicating with the physicians themselves.

Figure 2 shows another example of a virtual organization in a hospital. A 75-year-old man had a heart attack while driving and ran into a tree, broke his leg, had head trauma, and fractured his ribs resulting in a collapsed lung. A general surgeon was assigned who determined that the leg fracture was the least critical and recruited three surgeons: a cardiologist, a chest surgeon, and a neurosurgeon. As long as the leg was immobilized, an orthopedist was not yet needed. The general surgeon would supervise and determine the order of interventions including surgeries but would not do surgery himself or herself—this is the usual way a general surgeon works, supervising surgeons, most of the time not doing any of the surgery him- or herself (Goodman, 2007).

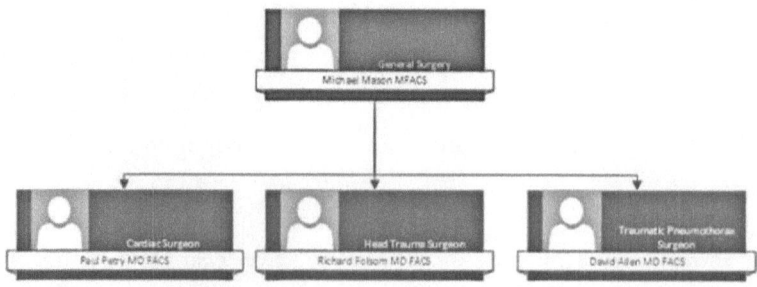

**Figure 2. Second Virtual Organization Example (Physician Names are Fictitious)**

I project that in the future, virtual organizations will be needed that include physicians who work in different medical organizations. Medical care is becoming so complicated that patients may need to go to remote medical organizations to get the proper care with follow-up care when they return home.

One of the reasons for this increased complexity is that diagnoses and treatments in the future will be at the cellular level, not just the tissue level, producing more categories of disease instead of one, resulting in greater specialization in treatment than today. An example today is breast cancer compared to what care was like in the past: whereas breast cancer used to be considered as a single disease, now it is many different ones (e.g., estrogen receptor positive or negative breast cancer, and progesterone receptor positive or negative breast cancer). One medical center may not be able to diagnose or treat these many new categories of disease. This process of finding more specialized categories of disease is referred to as *precision medicine* (National Library of Science, 2023).

In addition to these many new categories of disease, some medical procedures may be so complex that only a very few medical organizations may be able to perform them. For example, UCLA can use stem cells to treat some forms of macular degeneration (Bennett et al., 2014); if this is later commercially done, then it is likely this procedure could only be done at a few medical organizations in a country.

Thus, because of the future greater complexity of medical care, a patient may have to visit a remote medical organization to be treated. Further, that treatment may require follow-up care at the patient's home medical organization, and sometimes follow-up care may be so complex that the patient would also have to visit a third medical organization that is able to do the follow-up care but not the main treatment. This may involve physicians from several medical organizations who need to communicate with each other, and with some physicians who supervise the others. This is, in essence, a virtual organization across medical organizations.

# 12. Medication Management

Many patients, especially the elderly, take a large number of medications. Today, the patient's primary care physician is responsible for ensuring that the patient is taking the correct medications and that there are no side effects and drug interactions, but a physician may not be as qualified as an educated pharmacist to identify inappropriate medications, better medications and side effects and drug interactions.

The UPMR, and not any EMR, is guaranteed to have a complete list of a patient prescribed medications, although the patient may not be taking all of them.

I propose that in the future, by government mandate to control the current large government expenditures on drugs, a *consulting pharmacist* in the patient's home medical organization or connected with a utility EMR organization will meet periodically with all individuals who take a large number of medications. The consulting pharmacist will be disallowed from benefiting from the sale of medications to avoid a conflict of interest. Both before and while meeting with an individual, the pharmacist will be able to review the individual's mirrored UPMR and learn from physicians why they made medication choices and changes.

In this periodic meeting, the consulting pharmacist would identify any foods the patient eats or over-the-counter drugs the patient takes that could cause drug interactions or side effects; identify and record possible drug allergies; identify any possible drug interactions or side effects; make recommendations to physicians on alternative drugs that work better, cause fewer side effects or interactions or cost less (including non-medication alternatives); make recommendations to physicians on what drugs may no longer be needed; and advise physicians and the patient on any simplified schedule for taking the medications. On a confidential basis, with consent of the individual, a caregiver responsible for the individual taking medications could be involved in this process, especially in scheduling of medications.

An example of an individual whose life was dramatically improved by a change in medications was a developmentally disabled individual who could barely stand. After changing his medications, he could walk, run and live a much more normal life. Previous to this, physicians were giving medications one at a time without consideration of other medications, sometimes giving a medication to counter the side effect caused by a previous medication (University of California/San Francisco, 2015.)

Besides periodic review of a patient's medications, a consulting pharmacist might also review a patient's medications after discharge from the hospital. Patients are often prescribed new or additional medications when they enter a hospital. Especially for older patients, these medications may not be appropriate after the patient is discharged. Often, a patient's at-home medications are taken away and some may be re-prescribed; upon discharge, a consulting pharmacist may assist in restoring the patient's at-home medications (Parsons, 2020).

Besides review of a patient's medications, a consulting pharmacist could also receive a referral from a physician to review medications when the patient or physician has identified a possible medication side effect or drug interaction. The consulting pharmacist would then have a scheduled meeting with the patient, again with the consulting pharmacist having the patient's mirrored UPMR available. The consulting pharmacist should do research on possible side effects or drug interactions prior to the meeting.

As mentioned earlier, the secure healthcare network itself could warn a physician prior to a prescription of a potential prescription error. When a physician initiates the prescription of a medication for which the patient has a possible drug allergy, the physician will be told of this allergy. When there is a possible drug interaction with a previously prescribed medication, the physician will be told.

When a physician orders a prescription, s/he can also identify the number of refills and minimum period between refills. If any physician tries to order the same prescription within the refill period, the physician will be told.

A physician can terminate the existing prescription, which would probably most often happen if the prescription was not filled and reissue a new one.

In the future, when a physician prescribes a medication, she/he can associate it with a health problem and the medication will be recorded in the appropriate longitudinal disease history. If the health problem has been identified as having gone away, the physician will be given the option to terminate the prescription. Termination of a prescription can be done at any time with the consultation of the patient. A consulting pharmacist, when later consulting with a patient, could use this information to determine if the medication is appropriate to treat that health problem.

If a physician removes a medication that removal would be recorded in any associated longitudinal disease history

# 13. Quality of Life and Other Outcome Measures

Today, healthcare is measured at the macro level, not the micro level. In other words, it is unusual to measure the quality of medical care for a specific patient or the quality of medical care given by a specific physician. Instead, the healthcare industry is looked at, to determine if the current practices for a particular type of medical intervention (e.g., mammography) significantly improve morbidity or mortality. In the future, outcome measures will also be used to measure healthcare at the micro level.

*Outcomes* are ways of measuring a patient's health, especially after a medical intervention. Therefore, an outcome can potentially identify the effect of a medical intervention on a particular patient's health.

Some examples of outcomes are longevity, aka mortality (how long an individual lives after the onset of an illness or after a medical procedure for an illness) and morbidity (how sick the individual is after the onset of an illness or after a procedure). In the future, there will be greater use of a third outcome measure: quality of life (how disabled an individual is).

One example of a quality of life measure is EQ-5D (Brooks & Rabin, 2010) which develops a disability measure from 0.0 (total disability) to 1.0 (no disability) based upon 5 separate measures: mobility, self-care, usual activities, pain/discomfort, and anxiety/depression. This value can be determined from the individual; when the individual is infirm or young, it could be determined by a relative.

In the future, the quality-of-life measure will be recorded over the life of the individual. If the measure dips after a procedure or change of medication, then the procedure or medication could be causing a new health problem.

If the measure dips without any intervention, then the patient could be having a new health concern.

"Quality of life years," combining longevity and quality of life into a single measure, is abbreviated QALY. I feel that Americans place too much emphasis on longevity alone, ignoring quality of life. The QALY combines both longevity and quality of life into one measure. Consider the quality of life, say the EQ-5D value, measured over the lifetime of an individual as shown in Figure 3 where the quality-of-life measure has a value of 0.0 (no quality) to 1.0 (maximum quality of life).

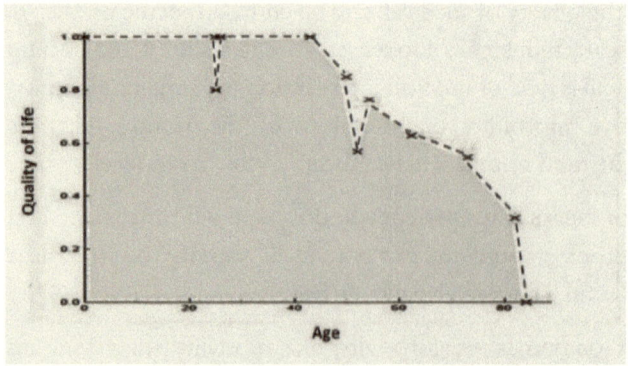

Figure 3. Theoretical QALY Graph

The QALY value for this individual is the area under the curve, about 70 years, although the person lived to about 84. This area accounts for an equivalent healthy time (of 70 years) during the individual's 84 years of life. The QALY measure ensures that longevity is not the only measure that is used, that quality of life is considered also.

The importance of using the QALY to measure quality of life along with longevity might be better elucidated in a second example. Consider a patient at the end of life with incurable metastatic cancer. The patient has a choice of either chemotherapy to possibly lengthen his life or a choice of hospice. Figure 4 shows an (entirely theoretical) QALY graph for each of the choices, choice 1 being chemotherapy and choice 2 being hospice.

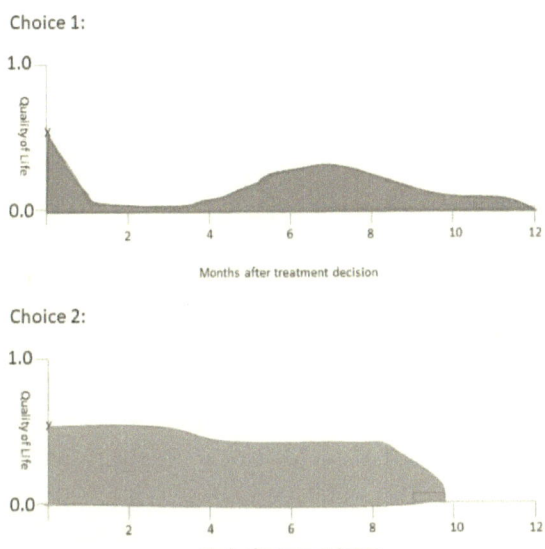

Figure 4. Theoretical QALY Graphs for End-of-Life Situations

In this theoretical example, the patient choosing chemotherapy lives longer, but the second patient's choice of hospice results in an overall better quality of life. Again, note that this is an entirely theoretical example, not taken from real life statistics.

Quality-of-life values, such as EQ-5D, could be recorded over time and included in the UPMR. Quality-of-life values could also be evaluated for a particular medical problem instead of overall, in which case they could be included in longitudinal disease histories.

For some procedures or injuries, pain, in addition to quality-of-life, measures could be recorded in a disease history after the procedure or injury. This information could be used in the research of how long it takes a patient to recover from pain that occurs after a procedure or injury, (e.g., how long after a knee replacement a similar patient no longer has any pain).

In the future, additional factors may be added to quality-of-life measures, beyond the 5 quality measures used by EQ-5D. For example, whether an extremely elderly person does or does not have a devoted caregiver has a big effect on quality of life. Also, there is an argument to be made that quality of life could be negative. For example, Vincent Van Gogh at the end of his life or someone trapped in the ICU on a ventilator at the end of their life might consider their quality of life to be negative and not worth living—this is an argument some use for euthanasia. But quality of life is more than how disabled you are. Quality of life for many people includes how well they are meeting their goals in life.

For example, a 50-year-old male with severe benign prostate enlargement may want to father a child. Having a prostate operation that destroys fertility may then have a different effect on quality of life for that male compared to one who does not want to father a child, even though they both could have the same disability rating—the same QALY graph using EQ-5D—after the operation.

The book *Achieving Your Personal Health Goals: A Patient's Guide* by James W. Mold, MD (Mold, 2017) argues that physicians should not only be measured by how many patient medical concerns the physician treats but by how well the physician meets the patient's goals in life.

An example is given of an adult patient who experiences some pain from a rotator cuff injury caused when he was playing baseball in high school. The patient indicates that the past injury does not cause him much problem, but he no longer has the strength to use a bow and arrow to go hunting for deer like he did earlier in life, a pastime he would love to restart. Considering the failure rate and long recovery time of rotator cuff surgery, the physician suggests that, rather than having the rotator cuff surgery, the patient could resume hunting again by use of a crossbow rather than the bow and arrow.

As another example, the goal of a terminally ill patient might be to be cognizant and be with his family during the remainder of his life rather than receiving a possible life-extending treatment that would destroy his cognition during recovery from the treatment.

A paraplegic with an incomplete lesion may have an initial goal of recovering the ability to walk the final few feet to receive her diploma.

Another individual may have the goals to walk without pain and to sleep at night without continually waking up.

A patient's *goals* could be included in the clinical summary.

Quality-of-life and pain measurements should be entered periodically, not just when the individual comes in for care. One possibility is to have the individual input these values, and when the individual does come in for care, move these values into the UPMR (including longitudinal disease histories).

# 14. Improved End-of-Life Care

One big problem at the end of life for terminally ill patients, especially in the United States, are treatments that provide little or no value and destroy the quality of life in the remaining days of the patient (Gawande, 2003). In the future, there will be a greater recognition of treatments that fall under this category. QALY measurements could be used by physicians to identify such treatments as not beneficial and hurting quality of life.

Apart from hospice care, longevity today is the main goal of end-of-life care rather than quality-of-life. There are a number of reasons for this. Firstly, family members not feeling the pain and anguish of the patient often would go to any measures to keep the patient alive. Secondly, American society considers it more horrific if an individual dies rather than is injured, say in a shooting, even if an individual is maimed for life and thus has miserable health; this is reflected in the severity of punishment for murder compared to attempted murder.

Another reason longevity is emphasized over quality of life is that an end-of-life patient may become too ill to speak for herself/himself and family members make decisions instead. For example, a patient's family could have the patient put on a ventilator to prolong her life, although she would not have previously wanted this. To take care of such situations, there are advance directives and POLSTs.

*Advance directives* and *POLSTs* provide guidance to medical professionals on the patient's care if the patient cannot speak for herself/himself. An *advance directive* describes care in hypothetical future situations; a *POLST* is similar but is a medical order developed by a physician talking to the patient based upon the current condition of the patient. POLST is an acronym standing for "Provider Orders for Life-Sustaining Treatment." A *healthcare proxy* names someone the patient trusts as the patient's agent to express his/her wishes and make health care decisions if he/she is unable to speak for herself/himself.

Sometimes a patient who cannot speak may indeed indicate by her/his actions that he/she wants to die or is ready to die. In two cases, I have had my dying relatives pull out their IVs and blood pressure monitors. Dying patients also often automatically refuse to eat. (I suggest that when a patient tries to remove IVs and other items that family members let them do so.)

Some states allow competent dying elderly people to request and receive euthanasia, which is a form of suicide. (Some Christians consider any form of suicide, including euthanasia, a sin as they view it as self-murder (Potter, 2021). I was told of a 100-year-old who was not terminally ill who chose, and the medical organization initiated, euthanasia; before he did so he met with each of his children, saying goodbye. It is likely that euthanasia will become more common, and accepted, in the future.

Hospice care does consider quality-of-life: Instead of being treated, a patient is given comfort care until her/his death. One problem with hospice care is there are no clear guidelines for when a person should be in hospice care and many individuals probably choose to go into hospice care too late in their lives.

An article in the NY Times by a hospice nurse, "How to Make Doctors Think About Death" (Brown, 2019), takes a different and more straightforward approach to preventing such non-beneficial treatments. She recommends establishing *guidelines for moving a terminally ill patient to hospice care*. The author of the article recommends the following guideline: "For patients who have one terminal illness that is either resistant to treatment or can't be safely treated, combined with a second very serious illness or complication, along with a high degree of physiological frailty, physicians should consider comfort care." This would be a guideline that all physicians should follow for end-of-life patients.

So how will end-of-life care improve in the future? I foresee the following:

1. Quality-of-life will become more important in treating patients at the end of their lives.

2. Family members will be advised by personnel who have had significant experience with end-of-life patients.
3. Clear guidelines will be made for when a patient should be moved to hospice care.
4. Patients will be given more flexibility in choosing euthanasia.

# ENVISIONING MEDICINE IN THE FUTURE

5.

# 15. Prevention and Self-Care Checklists

The *clinical summary* in the patient's UPMR contains next due and completed dates for preventive health interventions. The Affordable Care Act identifies these health interventions which insurance companies must provide at no cost. These include evidence-based screenings and counseling, immunizations, and preventive services for women (KFF, 2023). This chapter discusses preventive care more generally.

When providing patient care, a physician often meets with a patient for a few minutes. Within this time frame, it is difficult for a physician to convey information on self-care that a patient fully comprehends, and even if the physician does a good job of this, the patient is likely to forget much of the information. In the future, an approach to enable the patient to remember important self-care information will be a *self-care checklist*.

For an individual with a major but manageable chronic medical problem, it is much more productive to take measures to avoid medical problems than to treat them. A self-care checklist could identify a list of things the individual should do to avoid medical problems.

Identification of medical problems to avoid, given a particular medical condition, could be determined by looking at disease histories of patients who have had this medical condition. For example, a disease history for a paraplegic was presented in a previous chapter, a woman who had medical problems that are typical of many paraplegics:

1. Individual may not want to change
2. pressure ulcers
3. sepsis caused by a pressure ulcer
4. broken bones due to falls
5. blood clots

6. urinary incontinence.

A self-care checklist, then, for a person who just became a paraplegic would identify countermeasures to such problems, ways to avoid these problems during his or her lifetime (e.g., do lifts every couple of hours to avoid pressure ulcers, including when in bed sleeping).

Ideas in the self-care checklist could be reinforced by a nurse going over each point with the patient.

The process of identifying a countermeasure for every possible medical problem is very similar to what is done by nurses using a scheme for inpatients called NANDA. Nursing diagnoses (like our medical problems) are identified for the inpatient identifying medical concerns (e.g., "risk of falling," "risk of pressure ulcer," etc.). For each nursing diagnosis, NANDA identifies interventions to follow (e.g., for falling, "keep rooms free of clutter"). NANDA stands for North American Nursing Diagnosis Association (McFarland & McFarlane, 1997).

A self-care checklist would be developed for a patient by the patient's physician working in coordination with nurses. Besides identifying countermeasures for preventing medical problems, a self-care checklist should also describe situations where the patient should seek immediate medical care (e.g., if there is redness of the patient's skin indicating the start of a pressure ulcer).

Self-care checklists should be periodically re-discussed with the patient, with possible modification of the checklist to make it more up-to-date or more relevant to the patient.

In some cases, it may be useful to make the self-care checklist for both the patient and the patient's caregivers, potentially having the caregivers participate in activities on the checklist. A self-care checklist for a baby or child would commonly be developed for the child's parent.

The self-care checklist idea was an outgrowth of Atul Gawande's idea of having surgical checklists prior to surgery to ensure that the surgeon does not forget necessary activities prior, during, or after the surgery (Gawande, 2009).

In association with a self-care checklist, a physician could assign the patient with a class (e.g., what to do in preparation for a knee or hip replacement). When the patient must make a difficult lifestyle change, the physician could assign the patient to a health psychologist who would assist the patient in making the lifestyle change (e.g., to stop smoking).

Capitated medical organizations, rather than fee-for-service, would have more of an incentive for self-care checklists given fee-for-service organizations make more money the sicker you are. A capitated medical organization is one that gets paid an amount each month per member to provide comprehensive medical care.

MICHAEL R. MCGUIRE

# 16. Prevention and Health Psychologists

What is difficult for an individual is to change an ingrained lifestyle such as smoking, opioid use, prediabetes diet, anger, shyness, loneliness or lack of exercise. In the future, there will be *health psychologists* to assist individuals in making such difficult lifestyle changes. In the future, when a physician suggests a lifestyle change, the patient will also be assigned to a health psychologist.

A *health psychologist* is a psychologist who scientifically assists an individual in changing his or her lifestyle to live a healthier life and prevent disease—be the lifestyle change to stop smoking, stop taking drugs, revise a diet, get more exercise, manage stress, or other change. A health psychologist may also assist an individual in how to live with chronic disease (Taylor, 2015).

In the future, there will also be a greater number of employers who use health psychologists. Health psychologists will be employed to keep productive employees healthy, even in small organizations (which are more likely than large organizations to have employees whose loss would greatly hurt the company).

A health psychologist, like a self-care checklist, is especially useful for capitated medical organizations. A *capitated medical organization*, instead of only getting paid by insurers for fee-for-service, gets paid an amount each month per member to provide comprehensive medical care. Health psychologists would keep members from getting sick or keep members with chronic diseases from getting worse, thus saving money for the medical organization.

As noted earlier, in general, *fee-for-service medical organizations* do not benefit from programs that prevent disease—the sicker the patients, the more money the medical organization makes. However, governments who pay for medical care and individuals who could avoid a debilitating disease could benefit. Ensuring that fee-for-service medical organizations refer patients to health psychologists might require that there be a law to do so given certain circumstances (e.g., given that a patient has prediabetes and wishes to avoid diabetes or given that a smoker wishes to quit smoking, potentially later avoiding lung cancer).

Health psychologists will have the assistance of videos, classes and support groups both inside and outside the medical organization. For a health psychologist or support group to be of most benefit to an individual, the health psychologist or support group must not only provide general knowledge, but information tailored to the individual; for example, an exercise program with a personal trainer; a personalized diet plan developed by a nutritionist; or a detailed personalized smoking cessation program.

Health psychologists in a medical organization could have access to a patient's medical information in the secure healthcare network, including self-care checklists. Medical information could be used to identify whether the individual is prediabetic and allow the health psychologist to tailor a personalized program so the individual will not become diabetic. If an individual has injuries and it is a goal that the individual gets more exercise, an exercise program could be developed that does not aggravate the injuries. Like a physician, a health psychologist may also develop a self-care checklist for an individual.

In the future, health psychologists will be able to use the case (or episode of care) structure described in chapter 10 to manage on-going visits with a patient to prevent a disease or change a patient's lifestyle. As mentioned, diabetes is a disease that could be prevented for an individual with prediabetes through continuing care (Centers for Disease Control and Prevention, 2022).

The case structure would identify for a patient the health psychologist who is managing the prevention of the disease or change in lifestyle. The case would continually identify the next encounter to ensure that the individual comes in regularly for advice and moral support. The on-going care plan would be identified in the case.

This prevention approach has the potential to greatly improve the health of a population and to save significant amounts of money by avoiding debilitating and costly-to-treat diseases. A patient can avoid getting diabetes; a patient can quit smoking; or a patient can quit taking drugs.

There are obstacles to prevention programs and to attempting to change lifestyles:

1. No financial incentives for fee-for-service medical organizations to prevent diseases
2. Success of such a prevention program depends upon an individual's willpower
3. Changes in lifestyle are less possible without the support of one's family or friends
4. An individual might relapse in changing a lifestyle
5. A prevention program may require an individual to modify his/her schedule such as to miss work, which may result in the individual missing an appointment
6. Insurance companies may balk at paying when an individual is not sick.
7. Sometimes treatment involves treating the whole person; for example, a homeless person addicted to drugs may not be able to get off drugs until he can get a place to live.

These obstacles can be overcome by doing the following:

1. Requiring physicians in fee-for-service medical organizations by law to make referrals to health psychologists when prevention is beneficial
2. The health psychologist providing individualized advice including moral support
3. Including an individual's family members or friends in meetings with the health psychologist
4. Providing the health psychologist with a variety of support activities for the individual such as exercise programs and stop-smoking classes

5. Having the government pay for these prevention activities

6. Having the health psychologist be responsible for getting an individual in for care based upon encounter times that best fit the individual's schedule.

7. The health psychologist providing on-going visits with a frequency as necessary, allowing the individual to schedule another visit when the individual relapses

One lifestyle change recommended for patients by most physicians is restricting the amount of sodium (in the form of salt) in one's diet, as this decreases the chance of hypertension and cardio-vascular disease. What few physicians realize is that the ratio of sodium to potassium in one's diet is a greater predictor of disease, with a lower ratio being more beneficial and with most people consuming too much sodium and too little potassium (Vulin et al.,2022). The FDA is encouraging food-manufacturers to use potassium salt in place of sodium salt (Pugle, 2019).

# 17. Genetic Information, the Microbiome and Other Biomarkers

Along with the clinical summary, significant health problems and longitudinal disease histories, cases and episodes of care, and self-care checklists for a patient in the secure healthcare network, overall unchangeable biomarkers for the patient would be recorded along with biomarkers that are critical for the health of the patient. Again, a biomarker is defined to be a "cellular, biochemical, molecular or genetic characteristic or alteration by which a normal, abnormal, or simply biologic process can be recognized, or monitored" (McGuire, 2015).

Unchangeable biomarkers include date of birth and gender at birth. Such biomarkers kept for an individual could include genetic information. The microbiome, although it could be potentially changeable, could be included.

An example of a biomarkers that are critical for the health of the patient, and for all physicians to know, is that the patient has a pacemaker and the date on which consideration should be given to changing the pacemaker's battery.

The *microbiome* is all the microbes that reside externally and internally in a human.

Genetic information consists of the g*enome, mutations* and *epigenetic* changes. The *genome* consists of the sequences of bases within chromosomes that occur within the fertilized egg and are carried over to almost every cell in the human body. *Mutations* are changes in these bases that occur over time: errors that randomly occur when cells divide (which could result in a cancer). *Epigenetic* changes are changes in the genome not due to changes in bases (i.e., not due to mutations), mechanisms that turn a gene on or off without changing the cell's genetic code.

Both genetic information and the microbiome have been shown to be useful in medical care. For example, the genome has been shown to be useful in the dosing of medications; physicians look for mutations to tailor cancer therapies; and the microbiome in the gut could be used to identify a bowel disease.

Most importantly, the genome is used to identify genetic diseases including Down syndrome, cystic fibrosis, Huntington's disease, hemophilia, retinitis pigmentosa, BRCA gene induced cancers, some forms of Parkinson's disease, some forms of ALS, etc. A way to modify the genome in humans and other animals is CRISPR-Cas9; how useful this will be in medicine or how ethical this will be considered to be (whether in living humans or in embryos) will be determined in the future (Doudna & Charpentier, 2014).

As an example of the use of the genome for dosing of medications, there are two categories of drugs:

(1) *active drugs* that work before they are metabolized and (2) *prodrugs* that work after they are metabolized (Cho & Yoon, 2018). A physician prescribing one of these categories of drugs, to ensure the drugs work and do not have side effects, will adjust the dosage as necessary for slow metabolizers and ultra-fast metabolizers (as identified by a patient having certain CYP gene variants, genes that produce enzymes that control the synthesis and breakdown of chemicals in cells).

Given normal dosing, a slow metabolizer may get too large a dose of an active drug, while an ultra-fast metabolizer may get too large a dose of a prodrug. The milder narcotic codeine, a prodrug, metabolizes to the narcotic morphine; with normal dosage, an ultra-fast metabolizer could get a toxic dose of morphine (Sulakvelidze, Alavidze, & Morris, 2001).

In some cases *epigenetic* changes, events that turn on or off genes without affecting the genetic code, can be identified in an individual, such as extreme isolation when the person was young causing stunting of growth or deprivation of food for an individual's mother when the individual was a fetus producing later metabolic syndrome (Sapolsky, 2010).

(*Metabolic syndrome* is a combination of visceral obesity, abnormally elevated cholesterol in the blood, an abnormally high blood glucose level, and hypertension (Alberti, Zimmet, & Shaw, 2005)).

Another genetic biomarker is telomere length—the number of non-coding bases at the end of DNA, related to longevity. Telomeres shorten during cell division. Stress management and exercise are said to slow down this shortening (Blackburn & Epel, 2017).

Besides overall biomarkers, biomarkers specific to a particular disease may be kept providing information on how to better treat the disease; I call such biomarkers, *disease biomarkers*. Disease biomarkers will be transferred over from source documents to longitudinal disease histories related to the disease.

A disease biomarker for cancer may be the type of *receptor* inside or on the surface of the cancer cell. Any cell, including a cancer cell, may have *receptors* embedded in its cell wall or in the cytoplasm that bind hormones, neurotransmitters or drug molecules that together may have an effect on the reactions within the cell. Recognition of the type of receptor in cancerous cells could be important in the diagnosis, treatment and prognosis of the cancer.

Biomarkers will also be kept for interventions and other events within disease histories: predictive, pre-intervention and results biomarkers. These biomarkers will record results of interventions and enable prediction of the results and of future bad outcomes. Such biomarkers will be discussed in more detail in a later chapter on population research

# 18. Selectively Sharing Genetic Information

In the future, when the genome is available for an adult, say a person 18 or older, that adult can indicate that she/he wishes to share medical information with a close biologically related relative, given the relative's name and/or relationship. If the relative has the reciprocal designation and the system verifies through the genomes that the relationship does indeed exist, then sharing of medical information may be allowed. Thereafter, a physician caring for the individual will be able to see genetic information and significant medical conditions of the close relative in the individual's clinical summary. A sister may learn that the other sister has the BRCA1 or BRCA2 gene indicating that they each have a much greater chance of developing breast cancer than other women.

Communicating with relatives that they may share a gene variant that could cause disease is problematic. Maybe you do not want to share that information with other relatives. Maybe other relatives do not want to know about such information.

Medical practice may make more use of a person's genome in medical care in the future. Let us assume this will be so and that there is then the potential for one person to share matching genetic information with their relatives.

I propose the following:

1. **Relatives identified to share information with:** An individual can identify relatives with whom they would want to share genetic information by their relationships or names and relationships (e.g., sister, cousin, mother, etc.). The individual can indicate the specific gene variant to be shared or that the individual wants to share all genetic information that affects disease. The individual could indicate whether sharing the genetic information would or would not include the individual's name.

2. **Relatives indicate they want to receive genetic information:** Suppose one of those relatives indicated that they wanted to receive genetic information from that individual, categories of relatives, or all relatives. In that case, that relative could be informed of that genetic information. The individual could include or exclude categories of genes that they would like to receive information on (e.g., someone might wish to exclude genes related to dementia).

3. **Confirmation of relationships:** An analysis of the two individuals' genomes would confirm any specified relationship.

4. **Information shared:** The information would be shared with the relative only if there was a gene variant match in that relative's genome.

This proposal would allow an individual to share genetic information with selective relatives and ensure that the relatives would want to receive such information. And the individual could do this anonymously if they choose.

The secure healthcare network could use the patient's genome and search for other genomes where there is a required relationship (sister, cousin, etc.) and use associated UPMR information to identify names.

# 19. Early Treatment Diseases

Today, there is a disease that can be treated before it occurs: colon cancer. During a colonoscopy, polyps that could later turn into cancer can be removed.

Cervical cancer is also a disease that can be treated before it occurs. Cervical cancers can be predicted 10 years before a cancer may occur based upon analysis of a Pap smear of the cervix identifying precancerous cells. Precancerous cells can be removed by laser surgery and LLETZ (PBS, 2024; Prendville et. al.,1989).

There is also an existing blood test and clinical trials for a blood test to detect early stages of cancer (Cimons, 2024);GRAIL, 2024).

In the future, there will be more diseases that will be treatable before they occur. I call these *early treatment diseases*.

There are some diseases that currently cannot be reversed once symptoms are obvious— Alzheimer's is one of them. Other diseases may be treatable, but treatable with serious complications for the patient if they are discovered when there are obvious symptoms, and thus early treatment for these diseases might be useful also. I expect in the coming years that there will be research breakthroughs for many diseases showing how to predict the disease before it occurs, together with how to successfully stop the occurrence of the disease or to mitigate the disease upon its occurrence.

Much of the time this will involve molecular biology. Molecular biology potentially allows a diagnostic test to look at cells and identify disease pathways that could eventually result in the disease, and possibly allows a treatment that modifies the disease pathway, thus slowing or arresting the progression to the disease.

Even when there are such diagnostic tests and treatments for a disease, there could be several potential problems which could make early treatment difficult, including the following:

1. **Timing**: the timing of the diagnostic test and treatment may be critical for their success; if the diagnostic test is done too early, then it may be impossible to predict the likely future occurrence of the disease, while if the diagnostic test is done too late, the treatment may be too late to be successful.
2. **Diagnostic test complications:** the diagnostic test might cause complications. The diagnostic test might produce a false positive result and an unnecessary treatment might then be done, causing harm.
3. **Treatment complications:** the treatment may cause complications.
4. **Psychological issues:** the individual may not want to know the possibility that he will get the disease.

These possible problems complicate patient care: high-risk individuals may have to be selected and others excluded so that risks of the test and treatment do not result in overall poorer health of the community of individuals tested or treated. The individual may need to be brought in at the right time for the diagnostic test and then for the treatment. The individual must give his consent to the test and to the treatment.

For each such "early treatment" disease, an algorithm must be developed to schedule and control these events, which might include selection of candidate patients, consent or non-consent of the patient, and scheduling to bring in the patients at the right times for the diagnostic test and for the treatment

"Early treatment" is a completely different form of patient care than is done currently: not waiting until there are obvious symptoms before treating a disease.

# 20. Optimizing Physician Time Through Scheduling

It is estimated that in the future in the United States, there will be fewer physicians than needed to serve the population (Dall et al., 2024). To overcome or mitigate this shortage, physicians need to work smarter rather than work longer, as working hours could increase physician burnout.

There is a way to help physicians work smarter and be more productive: better physician scheduling. Such schedules would be relatively complex and require specialized personnel to create and maintain them, and to enable economies of scale, they would have to create schedules for many physicians.

I have been involved in the design of such schedules. These schedules have the following characteristics:

1. **Individual and combined schedules:** An individual schedule would be for a particular physician, facility, department or subdepartment and for a particular date. A physician could work in multiple facilities and multiple departments or subdepartments in a facility, so there could also be one or more schedules for a physician on a date. There would be a combined schedule for a physician for a date combining all his individual schedules. Each individual schedule would show the current state of appointments booked, time available for additional bookings, and time that cannot be booked for the physician on that date in the facility department,
2. **Time card:** A combined schedule could serve as a time card for the physician for that day.
3. **Non-bookable time:** a time period in a schedule identifying time that is not booked for appointments. Time seeing patients would be differentiated from time not seeing patients. A type code ending in '-' would indicate time not seeing patients (e.g., OFF- for off time or VAC- for vacation time) while a type code ending

in "=" would indicate time seeing patients (e.g., SUR= for surgery time.)

4. **Bookable time, a time for a potential appointment:** A bookable time in a schedule identifies a type of appointment that could be booked at a time in the schedule, with the time length of the appointment determined for that type at the department or subdepartment level. The type code for the bookable time does not end in a special character, with the type code identifying the type of appointment (e.g., URG for an "urgent" appointment or ROU for "routine" appointment.)

5. **Appointment search by type:** An appointment clerk or nurse could search for a particular type of appointment for a given facility, department or subdepartment and physician based upon time parameters such a time range, date range and day of the week; not entering the physician would search for available appointments for all physicians in the department or subdepartment. Up to three potential first-available appointments would be displayed at a time to allow the patient to make a choice; corresponding bookable times would be locked during this time to stop another patient from booking one of the appointment choices. The choice would create the appointment and remove the corresponding bookable time from further searches for available time.

6. **Bookable times over time converting to other bookable times:** General types of appointments are future (routine) appointments and same-day or next-day (urgent) appointments. The schedule would stack types so that if a potential appointment is not booked then the bookable time would convert to one or more other bookable types; for example, if a "routine" bookable time is not booked an identified number of hours before the date of a schedule, it might convert to two "urgent" bookable times, with the time for an urgent appointment being half the length of a routine appointment. An underlying bookable time is called an "alternate"; an alternate identifies the number of hours before the start of the schedule that the conversion would take place, with this conversion being done without human interaction.

7. **Some bookable times may not be available initially:** A bookable time may only be available for booking a certain number of hours before the date of a schedule. For example, an "urgent" type bookable time may only be available for booking a given number of hours before the start of the schedule, preserving that time period only for an urgent appointment close to the day of the schedule. Such a bookable time looks like an alternate having the number of hours before the start of the schedule that the bookable time would be available.
8. **Appointment search by time:** A nurse could search for available time in a physician's schedules or, by not entering a physician, in a department's schedules for the length of time identified by the type the nurse enters. A schedule would be shown having the available time length and the nurse could select to do the booking or to continue on to the next available time. The time required may consume one or more bookable times; booking an appointment would knock out all the overlapping bookable times. Before the search, like for a type search, the nurse could identify the patient's date and time availability. When the available time is displayed, the overlapping times would be locked from booking.
9. **A physician deciding to work harder during a certain time of day:** Either in the morning or afternoon, a physician may decide to work harder and see more patients. In order to allow this, "extra" times can be identified in a schedule to identify where another appointment could be made without affecting bookable time. A type code for an "extra" would end in a '+'; the type code is not used to identify the type of appointment booked.
10. **Appointment search for extra times:** A nurse—normally when a schedule is completely booked—could search for the earliest "extra" time in a physician's schedule or a department's or subdepartment's schedules. The schedule would be displayed with the earliest extra time, and the extra time would be locked from others. An appointment could be booked or the search could be continued to the next extra time. An appointment would not take away bookable time.

11. **Type search for a family:** A type search can be done given one or more patients, with the patients booked into a single bookable time. The bookable time would reopen for booking once all appointments are cancelled.
12. **Department searches:** When a search is made for all physicians in a department or subdepartment, then there must be no favoritism to selecting one physician over another, for example, physicians with names beginning earlier in the alphabet should not be favored.
13. **Booking an extremely urgent appointment:** A nurse could bring up today's schedule for a physician in a facility department and book an appointment at any time in the schedule. The nurse could identify whether the booking would or would not disable searching for the underlying bookable times.
14. **Display of a patient's appointments plus the ability to cancel an appointment:** An appointment clerk or nurse could display all the appointments for a particular patient. Any displayed appointment could be canceled, opening up bookable time that was disabled due to the appointment.
15. **Personnel creating or modifying schedules:** Parts of schedules, called "profiles," could be used to create schedules, possibly combining profiles to create a schedule. After creation or as part of schedule creation, a schedule can be modified, changing bookable, alternate. non-bookable and extra times within a schedule. Before a schedule is modified, the schedule is disabled from being booked. As part of modification or the whole of modification, a "hold" can be put over part of the schedule disallowing the time period from being booked further until the "hold" is taken off; in combination with the hold of a time period, all underlying appointments could be canceled.
16. **Schedules displayed during booking operations would look different than schedules during creation or modification:** During booking, non-bookable times, extra times, and currently non-booked bookable times would be displayed along with the appointments that were booked. During creation and maintenance, alternates all bookable times, including alternates, would be displayed.

17. **A physician becoming unavailable:** A physician may become unavailable, for example due to sickness. The schedule could then be held. Also, available would be the capability to transfer all or part of the physician's appointments to another physician's schedule. A list of cancelled or rebooked appointments would be created to enable a nurse to call up the patient.
18. **Releasing schedules for booking:** A schedule creator/maintainer, after the creation of new schedules in a department or subdepartment, could release the schedules for booking, beginning at the previous release through date and ending at a given date.
19. **Future appointments beyond the dates of available schedules:** A physician may want a patient to come in for a follow-up appointment at a date beyond the date that schedules are released, and so no follow-up appointment can be immediately booked. Information for a future appointment search by type could be saved for a patient that would result in an automatic booking when schedules within the identified date range are released; the patient would then be sent a notice of the appointment being made. I call this list of search parameters for future appointments, a "futures list."
20. **Reminder notice:** When any patient is appointed, the patient could decide to receive a reminder notice (email, text, phone call) shortly before the date of the appointment.
21. **Physician timecard:** Combined schedules for a physician can be used as a physician time card.
22. **Room and procedure scheduling:** This approach can also be used to schedule rooms and procedures.
23. **When a patient comes in for care, a visit is created:** When a patient comes in for care, the patient is registered and a visit is recorded.

The above approach to scheduling would have the following advantages:
1. This approach makes efficient use of a physician's time and works well with producing schedules with fixed begin and end times, e.g., for physicians working a standard work day.

2. The layers of bookable times would enable the mix of routine and urgent appointments to more accurately correspond to demand.
3. Urgent appointments could be made available for booking only at a time close to the start of the schedule.
4. The physician has control over when to work harder and see more patients.
5. This scheduling produces a "physician time card."
6. Extremely urgent appointments can be booked at any time with the option of taking time in the schedule or not.
7. A means is provided to handle physician unavailability—for example due to sickness—including the ability to transfer appointments to other physicians in the department or subdepartment.
8. Follow-up care for patients is enhanced, as the follow-up time could be at a date later than released schedules.
9. After booking, a patient could be reminded of the appointment, increasing the likelihood that the patient will show up for care.

# 21. Research

A *research database* will be a mirrored version of the total of UPMRs in the secure healthcare network together with the copies of associated source documents, except patient identity information will be missing from the database. The research database will thus be de-identified information; *de-identified* means all information identifying patients has been removed (McCallister, 2010).

The research database will enable *population research*, retrospective research of a large body of patient medical information. A problem with doing such research is that there is no guarantee there will be consistent data which will allow selection and comparison of patients as different physicians performing the intervention (e.g., a procedure) may decide to record different information.

To correct this problem, information collected in medical records could be made consistent by standardized collection of data for each type of intervention (e.g., each type of procedure) or for each clinical practice guideline. Alternatively, during patient care, lack of collection of standardized biomarkers in longitudinal disease histories would result in informing a physician that this data should be collected in the disease history (although it may not be in the corresponding source document).

Besides population research, another type of research is *a randomized control study* (Swinscow, 1997). This kind of research is done prospectively, set up before the research is done.

Because the experimenter determines what data is to be collected ahead of time, there is no problem in having inconsistent data. Risk factors for getting a disease can be determined whether or not the risk factor is currently tracked during medical care.

A randomized control study involves selecting patients who are appropriate for an experiment and randomly putting them in two groups: one where the normal approach is taken (a *control* group) and one where changed (experimental) approach is taken; and after the experiment comparing the two groups statistically.

Today, medical practice is restricted in how it can be performed. Various medical groups and the government create and store *clinical practice guidelines*, documents that describe evidence-based care and treatment for various medical situations. These guidelines could include alternative approaches to care. *Clinical trials* test out treatments that are not part of the guidelines, with successful clinical trials possibly resulting in changes to associated clinical practice guidelines. Prior to a clinical trial there may be medical research that forms the basis for the clinical trial.

There is a legal term used to determine if medical malpractice has occurred: standard of care. *Standard of care* is 'the level and type of care that a reasonably competent and skilled health care professional, with a similar background and in the same medical community, would have provided under the circumstances that led to the alleged malpractice " (Nolo, 2023). A patient signing an *informed consent* document does not override the need for a physician to follow standards of care.

A physician closely following clinical practice guidelines is safe from being below this standard of care.

One use of a randomized control study is to determine the effectiveness of a new proposed clinical guideline. For example, it was found that some cancer cells have *receptors* for estrogen on the outside of the cell. If estrogen molecules attach to these cells, the cancer increases in proliferation.

In the past, there was one clinical guideline for breast cancer. A new clinical guideline could be created for women who have breast cancers with this estrogen receptor. Drugs that suppress estrogen could be tested as a new treatment, producing a new clinical practice guideline for breast cancer patients having this receptor.

The medical community and government require that this new treatment go through clinical trials. Earlier clinical trials verify that the treatment causes no harm, while later ones determine the treatment's *efficacy*.

Doing these clinical trials involves a randomized control study. The experimenter finds women with breast cancer with the estrogen receptor who agree to the clinical trials. The women are randomly put into two groups, those who follow the current clinical guidelines (which at the time did not involve the new treatment), the *control* group, and those who receive the new treatment.

Women are randomly selected for the two groups to eliminate bias. Without randomization an experimenter might inadvertently select the healthier patients for the non-control group. If the experiment is completed, not finding toxic side effects of the medication, the results of the two groups are compared and it is statistically determined if the new treatment is better than the old one.

Note that this example shows the basis for *precision medicine*, changing medicine so there are more precise treatments for diseases.

# 22. Population Research: Prognoses and Selection of Interventions

A *prognosis* is "predicting the course and outcome of a medical condition" (Onisko, 2015). Today, physicians avoid giving a patient a prognosis for a medical condition, stating that every patient is different. In the future, with a comprehensive research database, a physician will be able to develop prognoses for the following:

1. **Determining if an intervention will be beneficial.**

2. **Predicting typical results of an intervention for similar patients.**

3. **Predicting the probability of a future outcome:** the probability of a future bad or good outcome occurring within a given time.

4. **Selecting the best intervention:** which of different possible interventions or a non-intervention would likely produce the best outcomes.

5. **Predicting what happens during recovery from an injury or procedure.**

## 21.1 Determining if a Medical Intervention is Beneficial

Today in the US, it is generally assumed that any medical procedure (or other intervention such as a medication) suggested or recommended and implemented by a physician for a patient is beneficial. (Further, through an *informed consent form*, the physician could be absolved of some liability if anything does go wrong.)

In reality, instead of a medical procedure always being beneficial, it may not achieve the desired results, and even if it does achieve these results, it may result in a bad outcome that is a side effect of the procedure.

Usually, the primary way to evaluate the procedure is to ask whether it significantly improves a medical condition or whether it stabilizes a worsening medical condition. A way to determine this is to record biomarkers before the procedure and compare them to these biomarkers after the procedure.

In the chapter on quality-of-life, Figure 4, an example—although theoretical—showed that performing a procedure at the end-of-life could result in a lesser quality-of-life for the patient.

Consider another example, a cataract surgery. Cataract surgery substitutes an artificial lens for the lens in an eye which has become cloudy with age. Assume now that there are many patients with disease histories for cataracts who have had cataract surgery.

For ophthalmologists to evaluate the quality of cataract surgeries, they might compare the following biomarkers before and after the surgery: 1) uncorrected vision and (2) corrected vision. A successful cataract surgery would, at the least, not show a degradation in these values. I call these sets of biomarkers recorded before and after the surgery, *pre-intervention biomarkers* and *results biomarkers* respectively. As it is undesirable to have results get worse over a given time after the procedure, another results biomarker might indicate the persistence of the results. Other results values are whether there were any complications because of the procedure, which I sometimes refer to as *side effects* of the procedure. See Figure 5.

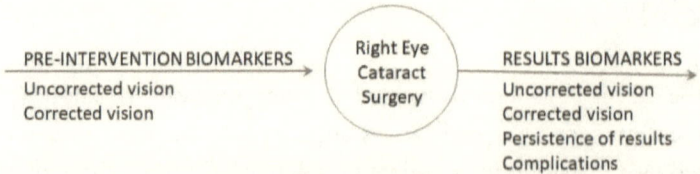

Figure 5. Biomarkers for a Cataract Surgery

The above two categories of biomarkers, pre-intervention and results biomarkers, would be included in any source document that describes a procedure, identifying biomarkers that could be used to evaluate the success or failure of the procedure with industry-wide agreement on what these biomarkers would be for a particular procedure. These biomarkers would be carried over to a disease history for cataracts.

Now consider the complications that could occur as a result of a procedure. I call complications of a procedure, *side effects* of the procedure. Two possible side effects of a cataract surgery are a *retinal detachment* and a *capsule tear*.

The *retina* (Wikipedia, 2023d) is "a light-sensitive layer of tissue that forms an inner coat of the eye." A *retinal detachment* (Wikipedia, 2023e) is "a disorder of the eye where the retina separates from the layer underneath." A *capsule tear* (Wikipedia, 2023b) is a tear to a "lens capsule that is a clear, thin transparent membrane that holds the lens within the eye," whether this is the original or replacement lens.

My ophthalmologist told me that with the level of myopia caused by my elongated eyeballs I would have a 5% chance of a detached retina because of my future cataract surgery. I trusted him that this statistic was true. To test this hypothesis, a study of patients having cataract surgery having the same axial length as mine could be done.

For each bad outcome, there is usually a *fallback position*. For example, for an unsuccessful hip replacement, you do it again. For an unsuccessfully treated detached retina, you still have the other eye. Unfortunately, I have severe macular degeneration in the other eye causing partial blindness, so I do not have this fallback position; I could potentially have become totally blind if I had a severe retinal detachment in the operated eye.

Assume that I do develop a detached retina after a cataract surgery. I then might have a (longitudinal) disease history for a cataract that looks like Figure 6. The diagram shows when the cataract in my right ("good") eye was first detected, when the cataract surgery occurred on that eye and its results, and when the retinal detachment occurred. Because the detached retina does not often occur immediately after the cataract surgery, the retinal detachment could have occurred due to the cataract surgery (say, with X% probability) or simply due to random chance (say, with Y% probability).

Section 21.3 provides an example showing how probabilities X% and Y% could be determined. Again, note that the retinal attachment associated with the cataract surgery most often does not occur immediately after the cataract surgery, but later (Olsen & Jeppesen, 2012).)

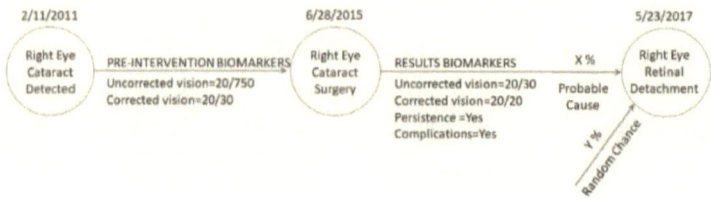

Figure 6. Disease History with a Detached Retina

## 21.2 Predicting Typical Results of an Intervention for Similar Patients

Medical research has identified biomarkers that determine the success or failures of an intervention. An assumption is that selecting patients who closely match your patient with these biomarkers will result in more precise predictions of outcomes of these interventions. On the other hand, using too many of these biomarkers may limit the number of selected patients.

Assume for the current patient, we want to predict what may be a typical outcome of an intervention based upon population research on similar patients. The procedure to do so then is as follows: (1) The selected patients have a similar past disease history up to the point of the intervention. (2) The selected patients have a similar set of biomarkers that predict the outcomes, which may include a similar age or gender. (3) The time frame to be studied has elapsed for the selected patients in the study, with the time frame long enough to include tested outcomes that do not occur after the intervention. (4) For each selected patient, it is determined what intervention outcomes have occurred.

As an example, say that it is now in the 2030's and we have many disease histories on cataracts. It is just before a female patient will be given a cataract surgery on her left eye and the ophthalmologist wishes to predict the results (outcomes by probability) of her surgery. Assume that it makes a difference whether the surgery is on the right or left eye.

Research (Desaia, Minassianb, & Reidy, 1999) and (Zare et al., 2008), has found that biomarkers that can predict the results of the cataract surgery are the following: (1) age; (2) gender; (3) axial length of eye; (4) glaucoma; and (5) diabetes mellitus. I call these *predictive biomarkers for results* of the cataract surgery. These biomarkers come from overall biomarkers in the UPMR (age and gender); cataract disease history (axial length); and significant health problems (glaucoma and diabetes).

As stated in the previous chapter, assumed biomarkers that measure the results of the surgery are the following: (1) uncorrected vision; (2) corrected vision; (3) persistence and (4) complications. I call the biomarkers measuring recorded before the surgery, *pre-intervention biomarkers* and those recorded after the surgery, *results biomarkers*.

See Figure 7.

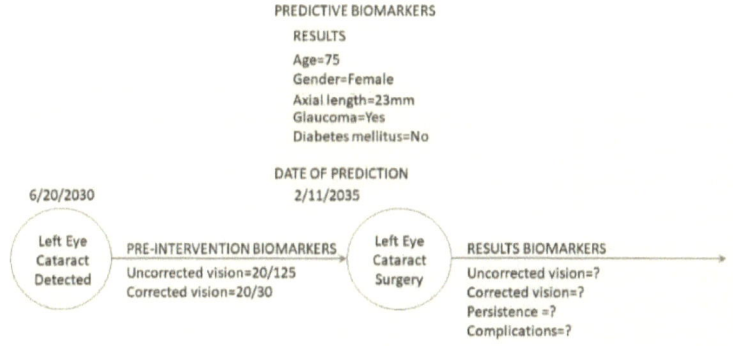

**Figure 7. Biomarkers for Predicting Typical Results of Cataract Surgery**

Individuals with a cataract surgery are considered for comparison to this patient. Those individuals with similarities of the pre-intervention biomarkers and with similar predictive biomarkers for results are chosen. Since we would like to predict persistence as well as complications, then only individuals with a sufficient time after the surgery to detect these conditions are chosen. These individuals' collective results after the surgery are then used to determine typical results for cataract surgery for patients similar to the studied patient. The studied patient does not have a detached retina prior to the surgery.

The results of this study would look similar to figure 8 with the exception that further analysis must be done to determine A% and B%. Instead, the study would only be able to determine (A+B) %. This further analysis is described in the next section

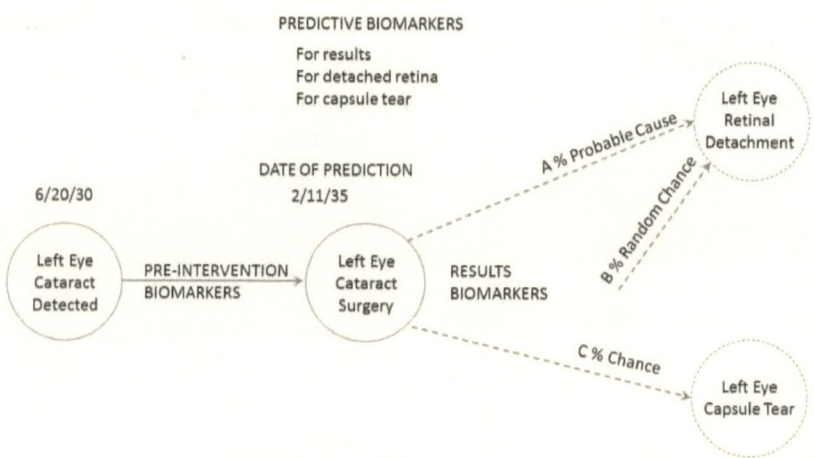

**Figure 8. Predicting Results of Cataract Surgery for the Patient**

Note that there could be too few patients selected to compare against the studied patient in which case the biomarker selection criteria need to be made less stringent.

## 21.3 Determining the Probability of a Future Outcome

As stated in the previous section, the analysis described can only determine the sum of A and B percent, the percentage of time a retinal detachment occurs after a cataract surgery. A further analysis must be done to determine B%, the probability that the retinal detachment occurred independently of the cataract surgery.

Say that doing the study of the effects of cataract surgery for a patient in section 21.2 that Z% of patients afterwards have a retinal detachment. If we do a study for a similar group of selected patients but who do not have the cataract surgery and find that Y% of them have a retinal detachment, then the probability of patients having the retinal detachment due to the cataract surgery is X% = Z% - Y%.

Note that some of the biomarkers used to select similar patients to the one studied may only be available when the procedure (e.g., cataract surgery) is done. In fact, axial length of the eye is only collected when there is a cataract surgery. In such a case either this biomarker must be excluded in both analyses or be replaced by a different related biomarker that has been measured for both (e.g., a measure of myopia).

A second analysis does not have to be done if the outcome can only occur after the cataract surgery. For example, the capsule tear only occurs because of the cataract surgery.

## 21.4 Selecting the Best Intervention

Two different types of procedures, or other interventions, could be compared for a given patient.

Say now that there are two different types of cataract surgery. Analyses of both interventions would be done for the patient. The ophthalmologist would probably pick the type of surgery where the patient was predicted to have the best results and the least combined chances of a retinal detachment and a capsule tear.

Besides comparing two types of interventions, an intervention can be compared to not doing the intervention. This is what was shown in Figure 4, comparing by quality-of-life measures, the effects of doing a procedure against not doing the procedure at the end-of-life.

## 21.5 Recovery from a Procedure or Injury

It is proposed that an individual record overall and significant health problem related quality-of-life measurements over time, even when the individual does not come in for care. These values would be transferred over to the UPMR when the individual comes in for care, including to longitudinal disease histories. Quality-of-like values, or pain values, could be included after an injury or procedure.

The latter would enable studies to determine how long it would take for a patient to recover after a surgery or injury, for example, when pain is likely to go away.

## 21.6 Ad Hoc Studies

Besides predetermined studies dealing with an event, ad hoc studies specific to a particular patient could be done. For example, since I have macular degeneration in one eye and the California Department of Motor Vehicles requires that I have 20/40 corrected vision or better in my other eye to drive, then a cataract surgery on that eye that resulted in corrected vision of less than 20/40 would have stopped me from driving.

Research has shown that a capsule tear during a cataract surgery results 30% of the time in vision that is correctable to a value no better than 20/50 (Chan et al., 2003), which is a vision level that would stop me from driving. Thus, it would be useful for me for someone to devise an ad hoc study to determine my probability of this happening.

# 23. Population Research: Accountability

As stated earlier, few medical organizations measure the outcomes of a physician's medical decisions and interventions. As a result, many physicians are not evaluated for the quality of their care and may not be held accountable for substandard care (Makary, 2013). In the future, each physician will be accountable for his or her medical care.

One way to do this is to evaluate outcomes of the procedures the physician has performed. This could be done for a medical organization, physician and type of procedure by looking through a time range of source documents for that procedure in the organization's EMR system. A longitudinal disease history associated with a procedure identifies the outcomes of the procedure. The percentage of different types of outcomes could be compared against all other physicians in the medical organization doing that procedure or against all physicians everywhere doing the procedure.

Physicians who perform high-risk procedures (e.g., cataract surgery for high myopia patients) should not be downgraded, as high-risk procedures are likely to overall have poorer outcomes. High-risk procedures should therefore be evaluated separately from normal, less risky, procedures

1. See Figure 9 for an example of an evaluation. In order to evaluate an ophthalmologist in the performance of non-high-risk cataract surgeries, procedure source documents within a chosen 5-year timeframe for all non-high-risk patients having a cataract surgery by that ophthalmologist are analyzed. The total number of cataract surgery patients since the ophthalmologist has practiced is also important, as this identifies how experienced the physician is in performing such surgeries. A physician can be compared against expected results determined either from all physicians performing the procedure in the medical organization or all physicians performing the procedure everywhere.

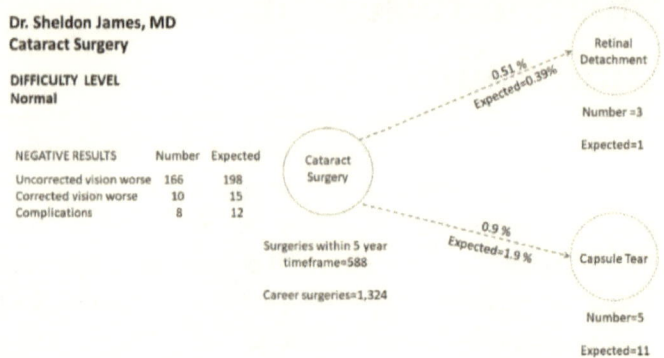

**Figure 9. Evaluation of an Ophthalmologist Doing Non-High-Risk Surgeries**

Such an evaluation of physicians performing procedures could be done just for the medical organization or to compare against all medical organizations.

This accountability information can be used in various ways, including the following:

- Evaluating the competency of physicians.
- Identifying physicians who need further training or mentorship.
- Weeding out incompetent physicians.
- Since physicians are expected to improve their skills with experience, identifying those physicians who are not improving.
- Identifying areas of weakness (e.g., excessive capsule tears).
- Enabling patients to pick physicians with experience and competency in a procedure, especially when a procedure is expected to be complicated.
- Enabling patients to select medical organizations based upon quality of care.

# 24. Complicated Medical Problems

*Pattern matching* is determining the diagnosis for a patient based upon previous patients presenting with the same symptoms, assuming the patient is like those other patients. When a patient with an unusual disease presents with different symptoms than normal, or has a different disease than originally expected, then the physician must go beyond pattern-matching and do an *analysis*.

Often physicians have little time to see a patient. As a result, a patient is sent to the assumed correct specialist. But sometimes the medical problem is so complex that it requires much *analysis* before the true nature of the problem is known and/or before the correct specialist can be determined.

In the future, there will be the following additional medical personnel for the more complicated problems that cannot be easily resolved without extensive analysis: a *physician consultant* and a *physician analyst* to analyze complex medical problems. The physician consultant will be people-oriented, spending most of the time interviewing patients, while the physician consultant will be more technically oriented, serving as a researcher and data analyst, although each will be equally knowledgeable about medicine.

Consider the following as an example of a complex medical problem they might try to resolve:

A middle-aged patient has recently fallen several times, often receiving significant bruises and twice breaking bones, once his left wrist and another time his right knuckle. The goal of the patient is "to stop falling."

He has an instep that sometimes weakens and becomes numb and knee pain, both causing him to limp. He has the start of cataracts and macular degeneration in one eye, and he regularly sees an ophthalmologist. Falling could have been caused by the patient's limp, by MS or other neurological causes, by a balance issue (such as an inner ear problem), or by a problem with eyesight. Alternatively, the falls could just be coincidental.

See Figure 10. Because the patient's primary care physician has limited time to see the patient and the patient has a medical condition that is potentially complex to determine, the primary care physician sends the patient to a *physician consultant*, who examines and interviews the patient, having time to do a detailed analysis of the patient's problem. The physician consultant has another person, a *physician analyst*, to do an even more thorough detailed analysis, including talking to specialist physicians and searching the medical literature. Together, the physician consultant and physician analyst develop a *game plan* for the primary care physician who can issue referrals for the patient to see applicable specialists. Part of the game plan is a later *follow-up plan* to ensure that the game plan was followed and that it achieved results or needs to be changed.

The physician consultant and physician analyst—upon interviewing the patient, reviewing the various falls and consulting with a neurologist for the limp and an ophthalmologist for a possible problem—speculate that an eye problem is the most likely cause of the falls, as the patient has often tripped over low benches and the patient has also expressed having problems with glare and driving at night. A possible problem is glaucoma which could cause loss of vision in the lower periphery of his remaining "good" eye as well as the glare and night driving problems; the cataract in his good eye is also of concern. The physician consultant sends a *game plan* to the primary care physician to refer the patient first to an ophthalmologist to give the patient a vision field test to look for loss of vision in the lower periphery with the option of the ophthalmologist to do cataract surgery on his good eye; afterwards, the patient will be referred to the neurologist. There appears to be no problem with the inner ear. The game plan also suggests that the patient see a podiatrist, who might correct gait problems caused by numbness in his instep.

The patient was indeed found to have glaucoma through the vision field test. Although this might not have resulted in all the falls, it was important to find this result, as glaucoma causes progressive untreatable blindness if not arrested. Glaucoma can often be arrested by eye drops. The neurologist also found a spinal stenosis which could cause the numbness in his instep, pain in his knee, and subsequent limp.

(Note that after having cataract surgery, the patient has not experienced any falls.)

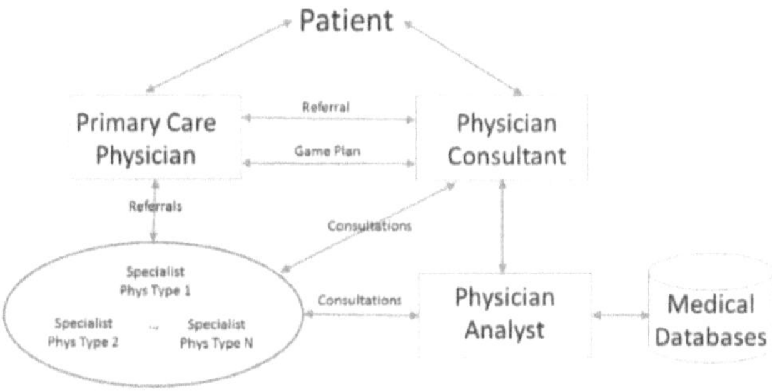

**Figure 10. A Physician Consultant and a Physician Analyst**

Besides providing analysis of complex medical problems, the physician consultant/physician analyst team will help patients select between interventions or non-intervention; this will be done upon request of a physician. After talking to the patient and using disease histories of similar patients, the physician consultant/physician analyst team will research alternative and new interventions for a patient's physicians to carry out, which could include clinical trials. The team will determine which interventions will likely produce the best results and fewest side effects using population research as described in chapter 20.

When necessary, biomarker values have not yet been collected, in which case the physician consultant will have the patient's physician issue medical orders to have tests done to measure the biomarkers (e.g., to do clinical laboratory tests).

Especially at the end of a patient's life, the physician team will advise the patient and the patient's family on whether quality of life is likely to be better or worse with proposed interventions, perhaps suggesting hospice care for the patient instead of any intervention. This would be suggested by differences in QALY graphs of similar patients having and not having the interventions.

Because the physician analyst is both a physician and technically oriented, he/she would be an appropriate person to perform another function: do the periodic reports evaluating physicians for the medical organization, such as was shown in Figure 9. This information would be available to physician management for evaluation of physicians and for accreditation of the medical organization.

This physician evaluation information could also be provided to patients. A patient could request a physician analyst to identify physicians who are best qualified to perform a high-risk procedure on the patient. For example, my ophthalmologist told me that cataract surgery for a person with my high degree of myopia has a 5% chance of resulting in a retinal detachment. The physician consultant could do a search of ophthalmologists that specialize in cataract surgery for high-myopia patients who have the lowest percentage of outcomes that result in retinal detachment.

# 25. Current Emerging Medical Ideas

The following are some major ways medical care currently functions that may become more prominent in the future:

- **Call centers:** provide telephone communication between a patient and an appointment clerk, advice nurse or advice physician.

- **Messaging:** the ability for a patient or medical personnel to send and receive back an email to and from a physician with the received email going through a nurse to prioritize the urgency of the response.

- **"Hospital at home":** providing acute care at a patient's home instead of in a hospital facility (Dressler, 2019, Winawer, 2018).

- **Telehealth:** a physician, physician assistant or nurse practitioner consulting with a patient and/or patient advocate via telehealth (telephone or teleconferencing) or observing a patient via telehealth as part of a hospital at home stay.

- **House calls:** visits to a patient's home by physicians, nurse practitioners or physician assistants—an idea from the past that is reemerging (Wikipedia, 2023c; Gordon, 2022)

- **In-home nurse care visits.**

- **Patient advocate:** a person who can help a patient navigate the healthcare system. Advocates ask questions, write down information, and speak up for the patient. They help the patient get the care and resources they need (CMS, 2023). (One idea is to have medical students serve as patient advocates for cognizant, but very sick, inpatients, so they can learn about the patient's point of view.)

- **Mobile medical vans:** mobile clinics or even mobile radiology (ANKE, 2023).

- Aging: It was thought that aging had to do entirely with accumulated mutations in cells, but Dr. David Sinclair of Harvard has shown that it is largely due to epigenetic (non-gene) changes, and he has shown that he and his colleagues can control aging in mice, even reversing aging and age-related conditions such as poor eyesight (Yang et. al, 2023). Dr. Sinclair thinks these ideas can be carried over to lengthening the lives of humans, making them healthier and even halting or reversing some age-related medical conditions. Billions are being spent on research in this area. (Park, 2023)

# 26. Revolutionizing Rural Medicine

Current problems with medical care in rural areas are the following:

- **Few physicians:** Patients in rural areas may not have quick access to specialty physicians or sometimes even primary care physicians.

- **Lack of medical facilities:** There may be few if any hospitals or clinics in the rural area and few buildings appropriate for clinics.

- **Lack of advancement opportunities:** It is difficult for rural physicians or nurses to advance in their professions, as they are isolated in a remote area.

- **Administration requires too much time and cost:** Medical organizations in rural areas may have to spend a lot of time and money on financial aspects of medical care, including insurance payments and payments to personnel.

- **Non-robust EMR systems, if any at all:** It may be too costly for rural physicians to have robust EMR systems if any, with EMR systems that are more dedicated to collecting money than to documenting patient care.

- **Variability:** Some rural areas have fluctuating populations—such as resort and vacation areas—and thus have a changing need for medical care and types of specialty care (e.g., orthopedics during ski and summer seasons). Also, rural areas, like urban areas, may have outbreaks of a disease that swamp the area's medical capacity.

- **Rural poverty:** People unable to pay for medical care.

In a large rural area where there may be many individual physicians or small medical clinics dispersed throughout, I propose a scheme where they could work together in the care of patients, a scheme I call a *medical alliance*.

Physicians and would each have schedules, with each schedule identifying date of the schedule, type of physician, the name of physician, location of physician, and for each appointment the time of the appointment, type of appointment (urgent, routine or either.)

An individual seeking care in the rural area would call into a call center. If the individual was seen before, s/he would have a list of past appointments. The individual would be told to call 911 in case of emergency. The individual could either make an appointment or talk to an advice nurse.

An appointment could be made for a named physician, or the earliest available of a type with additional options of finding the closest geographically and an additional option of AM or PM. For future appointments a date range can be entered.

Clinics and physicians in the medical alliance can share the same EMR services within a utility EMR system. When an individual is seen often by the members of the medical alliance, the individual can select to treat the medical alliance like his/her home medical organization, having a mirrored UPMR for the medical alliance.

The utility EMR system serving the alliance may have an office(s) in the rural area to support administrative services for the medical alliance, such as billing patients and paying physicians and clinics.

Another approach to providing care in a rural area is to have a large medical organization that has separate schedules for different facilities to treat the rural area like it had its own central facility (e.g., medical center) even though it does not. The medical organization could then be considered to have a *virtual facility*.

In some ways a *virtual facility* would be like a *medical alliance*, in particular the way scheduling of patients could be done, considering physicians and clinics that are closest to the patient.

But in other ways the *virtual facility* would be different. The virtual facility would use the EMR system of the larger medical organization, and if it is the policy, all patients would need to be members of the larger medical organization. Patients would have the larger medical organization as her/his home medical organization. The call center will function similar to a medical alliance, but also be able to appoint the patient with a physician located at other medical organization facilities, especially ones closest to the patient.

The secure healthcare network would treat a *virtual facility* as if it were an actual facility within the medical organization.

Currently, one downside of a physician being a rural physician is that advancement in the field is limited. For the case of a virtual facility, physicians in the larger medical organization could volunteer to spend a short time in the rural area, later returning to work in the larger medical organization, and thus have no obstacle to their advancement.

For example, a physician may be a skier and wish to spend the winter in a rural area that has skiing. Such rural areas that fluctuate in population could have physicians who work there when the population increases.

An alliance or virtual facility could also identify nurses and physicians who would visit your home, provide telemedicine, or a mobile clinic and ancillary services that could be brought to your home. For a virtual facility, physicians in its larger medical community could also provide telehealth and other services, including emergency and inpatient care.

An alliance or virtual facility could also provide nurses and visiting physicians for some patients who could be part of a "hospital at home" program, with the closest nurse and physician geographically to the patient assisting in the care of the patient.

A *virtual facility* is a way a large medical organization could provide care in an area without a large medical facility being there.

ENVISIONING MEDICINE IN THE FUTURE

# 27. Public Health

Public health will be more integrated with medical care in the future. Medical care will provide information to public health departments in real time. In turn, medical care will make use of public health information in patient care in real time.

When a patient has a new confirmed diagnosis for one of a list of selected diseases, public health agencies will be informed of the geographic locations frequented by the individual such as home, work or school. Public health officials will then be able to see a map showing the geographic locations and numbers of any listed disease, enabling public health officials to know where to concentrate their resources.

In turn, when a patient comes in for care with a complaint related to one of the listed diseases and the patient lives, works, or goes to school in a geographic location where there is a high prevalence of that disease, the physician will be told. This will enable medical organizations to use their diagnostic tests more efficiently, with tests resulting more often in newly finding the existence of a disease rather than being used mainly to confirm the existence of the disease for a patient with obvious symptoms.

Prior to the COVID-19 pandemic, a respiratory therapist told me that the pulmonary function test in his medical organization should be used more often to initially identify a patient with a respiratory disease, rather than mostly being used after such a disease was largely confirmed. If a patient comes in with shortness of breath and public health information identifies she lives in a neighborhood with a high rate of asthma, then that patient may be a candidate for initial identification of a respiratory disease via a pulmonary function test.

Public health will also be informed of selected diseases when they occur within a hospital, so that public health can identify the outbreak of that disease in a hospital. The hospital administration will also be informed.

When a physician identifies that a food product caused food poisoning, the identity of the food product if it can be determined will be sent to public health. Also, public health will be informed of the likely restaurant where the food poisoning occurred or the store where the food product was bought. Public health would then be able to more quickly stop an epidemic.

Some diseases of significance cannot be diagnosed. In such a case, public health will receive a report on the disease based upon its main symptoms. This may allow public health to identify an outbreak of a rare, seldom seen, disease if it receives multiple similar reports.

# 28. Confirmed Diagnoses

For medical information to be most useful for research, it should record confirmed diagnoses—not just tentative and differential ones—and identify them as such. Sometimes adequate care can be given based upon a differential diagnosis as the same care may be provided for a broad category of similar diagnoses.

Although it is important for each medical condition identified in a longitudinal disease history to have a confirmed diagnosis to support research, it is also useful to include the patient's complaint and differential diagnoses that have been ruled out or are currently in question which could lead to the confirmed diagnosis. The tests and procedures that are used to test the diagnoses should also be included. I call this string of the complaint, differential diagnoses, and tests and procedures a *roadmap* leading to verification of the confirmed diagnosis.

Within a disease history, roadmaps and the confirmed diagnoses should be clearly identified so differential diagnoses can be distinguished from confirmed diagnoses. Evaluation of outcomes should be based upon confirmed diagnoses and not differential ones.

An example of a patient complaint is "continual mucus in the esophagus." Differential diagnoses to be tested could include GERD, sinusitis, allergies, and bronchitis, among others.

"Roadmaps" are useful to enable later evaluation of the early part of patient care and to identify the probability of a given confirmed diagnosis given a specific category of patient complaint.

Testing of differential diagnoses, and thus a roadmap, could occur over one encounter or many.

One problem with "big data," using source documents for data analysis, rather than using disease histories is that source documents cannot be changed once signed off and they often only contain differential diagnoses whereas a (longitudinal) disease history can be later changed to include the confirmed diagnosis which might be determined later.

# 29. Patient Mirrored UPMR Access, Auditing and Data Analysis

Direct access to the UPMR is limited to specific EMR users to protect against hackers. A mirrored copy of a patient's UPMR will be available at each medical organization that is a patient's home medical organization; a mirrored UPMR is considered to be a medical organization database and access to it if allowed by the medical organization would be controlled by medical organization security measures. Although it can be read, the mirrored UPMR is not available for change by the medical organization.

Without an existing UPMR, many medical organizations today currently display a patient's medical information to the patient over the Internet using security governed by the medical organization. A medical organization can likewise display a patient's mirrored UPMR database to the patient over the Internet using the medical organization's security measures. This approach disallows Internet access to the UPMR directly from the secure healthcare network.

With the assistance of a *physician consultant* and *physician analyst* an individual could also do independent research based upon the patient's mirrored UPMR database and the research database. The patient would need to go to the utility EMR organization or his/her home medical organization after scheduling time with the physician consultant. The patient could do population research like what is described in chapters 20 and 21. The physician consultant interviews the patient, the physician analyst does the research, and the physician analyst later reviews research results with the patient. The physician consultant can order any tests for the patient to gather any necessary biomarkers for the data analysis.

Another service of a physician consultant is auditing information in the patient's UPMR with the patient. If any changes are suggested, this information would be sent to the patient's primary care physician to update the UPMR through the EMR system.

# 30. Increased Use of Artificial Intelligence

In general, based upon subject matter entered by a user and a large amount of related information outside the user, an *artificial intelligence (AI)* program produces an analysis in readable form, simulating results that could have been produced by an intelligent human being.

AI programs in medicine are computer programs that assist a physician (or an individual) in the diagnosis or treatment of a medical condition or support a physician or nurse in documenting medical record information. There will be much greater use of artificial intelligence programs in the future.

Google AI Mode and ChatGPT™ (Baker, 2023) are chatbots, general purpose AI programs that allow a user to get information on a topic from massive amounts of information, bringing back summary information in readable form. They use a large language model (LLM) to create a readable summary of information. These programs can be used both by physicians and patients to gather information on medical topics, in particular on rare diseases not often studied in medical schools (Wojtara et. al, 2023). For more ideas on ChatGPT for medicine, see (Pearl, 2024).

One program used by individuals is the Apple watch, which can identify atrial fibrillation in the wearer (Pepplinkhuizen, et al., 2022), which significantly increases the risk of the individual getting a stroke. So far, an Apple watch cannot identify a heart attack or a stroke (Apple, 2024).

Such programs are called "monitoring programs." Data is gathered from the individual real-time and analyzed for an abnormal medical condition. When the monitoring is done by a medical organization, there is often so much information that is needed to identify an abnormal situation that medical organizations are hesitant to do monitoring. For example, my medical organization monitors everyone with pacemakers, but only analyzes the information if the patient phones in a problem, as actively analyzing all monitored data for the 2000 patients with pacemakers in the region is not feasible.

One of the first artificial intelligence programs was MYCIN (Buchanan & Shortliffe, 1984), a program which chooses therapies for patients with infections. It was criticized for being a "black box," a program that physicians did not understand how it worked. This is still a criticism of most artificial intelligence programs that provide diagnostics, but this could be a problem: if something went wrong, then the user would not know what to do to fix the problem.

For example, I took home a machine that I attached to myself when sleeping to test for sleep apnea. It attached a sensor to my sternum which recorded vibrations. I accidently turned on my cell phone to listen to music and put it on my sternum. I was concerned that it affected the results of the analysis, and I included a note with the machine.

Because the medical organization did not know what to do, if anything, to fix any bad results, they just accepted the results as is. Perhaps they should have had me redo the test.

Another type of artificial intelligence program is one that learns to do diagnosis by being given many examples of patient data and for each is told a physician-determined correct diagnosis based upon physician analysis of the data. Later, given similar patient information, the program then can make a diagnosis on its own. For example, the program is given diagnostic images of female breasts and with each radiologist's analysis of whether cancer is present; after being trained, the program can then do analysis on its own.

Applicable areas where this approach is useful are radiology, pathology, ophthalmology, pulmonology and cardiology (Ahuja, 2019), and septic detection (Young, 2024). An example of AI in both pulmonology and cardiology is the interpretation of stethoscope sounds (Littman, 2020).

It has been shown that the human radiologist analyzing diagnostic images for breast cancer has a 6% error rate including false positives and false negatives (Ahuja, 2019). Theoretically, if the artificial intelligence program instead is trained on actual outcomes (e.g., biopsies of breasts to determine if a woman indeed has cancer), then the artificial intelligence program could do better than 6%. This book shows a way to have a large research database, enabling an artificial intelligence program to have a larger number of outcomes and thus outcome-based learning examples than currently.

Now AI, say for analyzing mammograms, could do potentially worse than human physicians, the same or better, but sometimes the choice might go beyond a binary one (that a woman has breast cancer or not.) A woman with proliferative breast lesions is often reported by humans as having breast cancer when she does not have it, a false positive. However, such lesions could go on to breast cancer and removing them could forestall the future occurrence of cancer (Brett, 2024). An AI program correctly reporting she does not have cancer would not proceed to having a physician decide to do this procedure. (Note that this is another case of an early treatment disease.)

If artificial intelligence takes over for radiologists in detecting breast cancer, then fewer radiologists might then have the ability to do this analysis. A radiologist could potentially justify why he/she made a diagnostic decision, whereas the artificial intelligence program based upon pattern-analysis would not.

There are other types of artificial intelligence programs.

There is at least one robot: the da Vinci surgical robot assists the surgeon in treating a patient enabling surgery to be done with greater intricacy and precision (Fresch, et al, 2013). In the future will a robot be able to perform a surgery itself without surgeon intervention ().

AI can also be used to create SOAP notes from verbal inputs of physicians or nurses and to create hospital discharge summaries based upon documentation created during an inpatient stay.

Today, the large amount of medical documentation that a physician or nurse enters during point of care distracts from patient care. A new type of AI purports to automatically create EMR information from the physician's or nurse's conversation with the patient during point of care. Some examples are *Freed* ™ *and Deepscribe* ™.

At UCSF discharge summaries created by physicians were compared with AI-generated discharge summaries. It was found that ones created by AI were comparable to those created by physicians. UCSF recommended that the AI generated version be used as a draft and be updated by the physician (AI Brew, 2025).

AI can also be used to support capabilities proposed in this book.

If a new health problem is reported by a physician, then a new longitudinal disease history would automatically be created for it. A physician can identify that an encounter is associated with one or more health problems; the AI program will identify what information is to be added to the disease histories for these health problems.

When a procedure has the possibility of causing a bad outcome and that bad outcome occurs, then that bad outcome should be included in any longitudinal patient history containing that procedure. For example, as presented earlier, a cataract surgery can increase the probability of the patient having a detached retina. So, if a detached retina occurs after a cataract surgery, it should be included in a disease history for the health problem being tracked as well as adding the new significant health problem of a detached retina.

The research database, mirrored UPMR medical information for the patient, and general medical knowledge could be used together to analyze the patient's medical situation and do population research to make recommendations on diagnosis and future care. As an alternative to a physician consultant and physician analyst doing this research for a patient or physician using database analysis, a dialog could be set up between the patient or a physician using a chatbot to do this research.

See chapter 23 on physician accountability. Some AI systems make recommendations in appropriate circumstances (Littman,2020). Based upon research identified biomarkers, an AI program can identify a difficult procedure, one that has a high probability of having unfavorable outcomes. Based upon the evaluation of physicians in a department performing the procedure, the expertise of the physician in avoiding these unfavorable outcomes can be determined. The AI system could recommend that the difficult procedure be assigned to a physician with higher expertise or that such a physician assist the lower-expertise physician. The AI system could alternatively recommend that a lower expertise physician get training in a specific procedure skill.

As stated earlier and shown by the above examples, AI has the potential of freeing physician time and producing large cost savings for a medical organization. Professor Aymeric Lim, the CEO of National University Hospital in Singapore said, "Every healthcare system in the world has the same challenges, which are rising costs, an aging population and a decreasing workforce" (Young, 2024).

A big potential problem with AI is that it could take a physician out of the loop, and then there would be no one to identify when AI went wrong (Young, 2024)

ENVISIONING MEDICINE IN THE FUTURE

# 31. Precision medicine

Today, disease diagnosis is mainly at the tissue level (skin, lung tissue, liver tissue, etc.). In the future, diagnosis will be more and more at the cellular level, looking inside and at the boundaries of cells. This will enable *precision medicine*, producing more tailored and effective treatments.

Within cells, whether these are normal or cancerous human cells or cells of bacteria, there are chemical reactions that occur controlled by the cell's external environment. A cell has *receptors* embedded in its cell wall or in the cytoplasm that bind hormones, neurotransmitters or drug molecules that together may influence the reactions within the cell.

When medical care is at the cellular level instead of the tissue level, then a disease that today may be viewed as one disease may in the future be viewed as several different diseases. For example, breast cancer cells have recently been categorized by the type of receptors on the outside of the cancer cell, with the disease "breast cancer" now being treated differently based upon the receptors (estrogen-positive or negative, progesterone-positive or negative, and HER2-positive or negative receptors).

For a particular cell type, the set of external actions together with the internal chemical reactions that occur within a cell that eventually result in each disease are referred to as *disease pathways*. For example, frontotemporal dementia is known to have three different disease pathways. It is then possible that there could be three different treatments for the disease, with the treatment tailored to the pathway (Kandel & Rose, 2012).

Genes within the DNA in the nucleus of a cell also influence internal chemical reactions in the cell. The DNA (in chromosomes) in all the cells in an individual's body has essentially the same set of genes apart from mutations. A person's particular genes may influence patient care and treatment of a disease. For example, it is known that a woman with a particular BRCA1 or BRCA2 gene variant has a much higher risk of getting breast cancer, and her disease may have to be treated differently than for women without the gene variant, as her cancer is likely to be more aggressive (Smith, 2011).

This discovery of differences at the cellular and gene level will result in medicine that is more tailored to the individual, requiring not treating a broad disease category (e.g., breast cancer), but treating a more specific disease category (e.g., estrogen- positive breast cancer or BRCA2-breast cancer). This subcategorization of diseases will result in some current disease classifications to be too broad and will require additional biomarkers to identify the disease—I call these additional biomarkers to identify a disease together with current biomarkers of the disease, *disease biomarkers*.

There will be greater use of *precision medicine* in the future. There will be new mechanisms to support precision medicine, as precision medicine is likely to differ from current medicine in that (1) it will require super specialization of care; (2) it is more likely to require care at a medical organization or multiple medical organizations outside your own; and (3) it may require later follow-up care with physicians at the patient's home medical organization coordinating with physicians at the outside medical organizations. A medical organization providing very specialized care, being the only one or one of a few such medical organizations providing this care, I call a *center of medical expertise*.

A virtual organization of physicians—some at the patient's home medical organization, some at the center of medical expertise, and some possibly at a third medical organization--could facilitate communication required for the follow-up care.

# 32. Searching for a Medical Service

Today, medical services for a patient are largely at the patient's home medical organization or at a location geographically close to the patient. When services are not available locally, the patient may be sent to a medical organization outside the patient's geographic area.

In the future, there will be greater support for finding the most appropriate available medical service for a patient no matter where it is located. Some upsides of doing this are the following: (1) a patient could receive a medical service unavailable in the patient's geographic area; (2) interventions could be selected based upon the specific characteristics of the patient, providing support for precision medicine; (3) a physician could be selected to do a risky procedure who has the highest competence in doing this type of procedure; (4) interventions could be selected based upon their cost, saving the patient money; (5) medical organizations could make better use of their otherwise underused resources (e.g., MRIs that are otherwise underused or physicians who treat rare diseases and who would otherwise get few patients).

There will be a catalog of medical services in medical organizations for patients, with the catalog available to physicians. Services will include *clinical trials*. The physician can select a service for a patient, in some cases being able to directly schedule an appointment for that service.

Any medical organization could be included in the catalog with the catalog identifying (1) the name and a description of the service; (2) the criteria for the patient to be eligible for the service, which could include a list and range of biomarkers that a patient must possess to be applicable for the service; (3) the geographic location where the service or preparatory activities would be performed or an indication that the service could be provided through telemedicine; (4) the benefits and risks of the service; (5) optionally, the cost of the service; (6) optionally, the physician performing the medical service and an evaluation of the physician's performance providing the service; and (7) contact information for the service.

A physician could search through the catalog based upon various criteria, including (1) the type of service, optionally including patient biomarkers related to the service; (2) the geographic location of the patient; (3) an indicator that cost is of consideration; and/or (4) an indicator that experience or expertise in doing a specific medical service is a consideration. Search results would be returned in the most appropriate order (e.g., closest geographic location, least cost, highest expertise, closest match to biomarkers).

Besides a patient's physician, a physician consultant and physician analyst could use this search. They would likely use this search most commonly to (1) search for alternative interventions applicable for a patient or (2) search for a physician who has the most experience or has the highest competence in performing a high-risk procedure.

In some cases, direct scheduling of the medical service may be allowed when a physician finds a service through the catalog. After finding a service that is applicable for a patient, the physician could search for an appointment for that service based upon date/time parameters identifying when the patient is available. A list of available appointments would be displayed, and the patient could select one.

For complicated services, instead of providing a means to schedule the service, a meeting with the patient would be provided to determine if the patient met the criteria for the service first. Medical organization(s) might contract with the medical organizations doing the procedure to do the pre-screening.

This approach could prevent a center of medical expertise from being inundated and could result in some patients not having to travel so far away from their homes to have the screening.

Once a visit has been set for the patient for the physician's service or set up to evaluate whether the patient is appropriate for the service, the patient's physician could issue an *outside medical organization referral* to that physician. This would be done with the authorization of the patient. Afterwards, the referred-to physician would be allowed to see the patient's complete medical information through the secure healthcare network.

MICHAEL R. MCGUIRE

# 33. A Projected Example of Precision medicine in the Future

*Precision medicine* (in the past called *personalized medicine*) is a type of medical care in which treatment is more customized to the individual patient by performing medicine not only at the tissue level, but at the cellular level, the latter of which would provide additional information for diagnosis and treatment of the disease. In the future, precision medicine will be more commonly practiced.

In the future, it will be more common that a particular precision medical procedure, due to its complexity, will only be done at a few medical organizations in the nation. And it is possible that only a selected few patients would be candidates for the procedure.

Consequently, I foresee that in the future that medical organizations doing the procedure will form contracts with a larger number of other medical organizations throughout the nation to evaluate patients as candidates for the procedure. The selected patients would then be able to contact the medical organization doing the procedure to get an appointment to do the procedure.

This approach has the dual advantages of (1) having the potential patients travel shorter distances for screening rather than traveling to the performing medical organization, which is likely to be further away, and (2) allowing the medical organization doing the procedure to deal with a smaller number of patients.

Consider a current experimental procedure that is done for macular degeneration at UCLA (Bennett et al., 2014). UCLA today performs an experimental procedure for treatment of macular degeneration that is related to the dying of retinal pigment epithelium (RPE) cells, cells that provide nutrition for light-sensitive photoreceptors in the eye. The procedure involves modifying human embryonic stem cells in the lab and turning them into RPE cells. The cells are then injected into the patient's diseased eye. Some patients have received significant improvement in vision. (The eye is one area of the body that does not produce a strong immune response due to the blood-brain barrier.)

Say that this treatment advances beyond a clinical research study and is performed both in Los Angeles and Boston. And imagine that potential patients must first be screened to determine that they are appropriate candidates for the procedure, with this evaluation occurring in 20 different geographic locations in the United States. This evaluation for appropriateness of RPE treatment for macular degeneration could be included in the online catalog.

Using the catalog, an ophthalmologist with a patient who has macular degeneration could look up treatments for macular degeneration, finding this stem cell treatment for macular degeneration along with requirements for the procedure, and the benefits and risks of the procedure. The ophthalmologist could enter biomarkers for the patient to determine if the patient qualifies for the procedure. The ophthalmologist could consult with the patient to determine if the patient would be interested in the stem cell treatment, explaining the ramifications.

If the patient was interested in having the procedure, a search could be made by the ophthalmologist through the catalog to find the geographically closest medical organizations doing an evaluation which had openings. If the evaluation facility allowed booking through the catalog, then a patient could be directly booked with the evaluation facility; otherwise, the patient would have to contact the facility to make the appointment. With the authorization of the patient, the patient's ophthalmologist would then send a referral to the organization that would allow the physician receiving the referral to see the patient's complete medical information through the secure healthcare network.

The patient would then go to the evaluation facility. A health care advisor at the facility would describe the macular degeneration procedure in detail, including the benefits and risks. If the patient agreed to the procedure, an evaluation of whether the patient was a suitable candidate would be done.

Upon the patient's return from the evaluation facility, if the organization determined that the patient was an appropriate candidate for the stem cell procedure and one or more of the treatment locations had openings, the patient would be contacted by a treatment location and told of the openings. If the patient accepted the opening, the patient would be asked to have his ophthalmologist send a referral to the treatment organization, allowing a treatment organization physician to also see the patient's complete medical information.

The patient would show up for treatment at the appropriate time. Prior to the procedure, the patient would meet with the treating ophthalmologist to again learn of the procedure's benefits and possible complications. The patient would sign a consent form and the stem cell procedure would be done.

Since this stem cell procedure likely has a risk of going wrong after the patient returns home, the ophthalmologist at the treatment facility might set up a virtual organization for the stem cell treatment, with the treatment ophthalmologist represented by an episode of care and the home organization ophthalmologist represented by a case or another episode of care lower in the hierarchy, as the home ophthalmologist may require later supervision from the treating ophthalmologist in providing follow-up care. After the patient returns home, any patient encounter dealing with the procedure would be communicated back to the ophthalmologist at the treatment organization as a feature of the virtual organization. This would not substitute for direct communication between ophthalmologists, but could facilitate such communication, especially dealing with any complications of the eye procedure.

Sometimes the care that is needed after the patient leaves the medical organization performing the procedure will be so complex that it cannot be done at the patient's home medical organization. In such a case, the performing medical organization might again contract with medical organizations throughout the nation to do this follow-up care, providing the patient with a means to get this care without needing to go a long distance back to the performing facility.

# 34. Design Choices, Alternatives and General Issues

This chapter describes design decisions made in this book and why they were made, concerns, and alternative choices:

1. There will be two categories of EMR systems, (1) stand-alone EMR systems, and (2) utility EMR systems that provide EMR services to many medical organizations. This enables all medical organizations, including smaller ones, to have EMR capabilities and limits the number of connections between EMR systems and the secure healthcare network.
2. Connections between EMR systems and the secure healthcare network are point-to-point and not through the Internet. This disallows Internet hackers from accessing UPMRs.
3. All EMR systems are large-scale with built-in software designed by the manufacturer, not software built by others. This allows EMR systems to be vetted for security leaks.
4. A UPMR for a patient is built from EMR inputs from medical personnel providing care for the patient.
5. The UPMR for a patient is only available for view in an EMR system to (1) an EMR user at the patient's "home medical organization;" (2) an EMR user at another medical organization if the patient is at the medical organization and provides biometric information to identify himself or herself; or (3) an EMR physician receiving a referral from a physician who is in category (1) or (2). This limits unauthorized access from people in other medical organizations.
6. What are the criteria for assigning a home medical organization to an individual? What are the criteria for removing a home medical organization designation from an individual?
7. There will be a mirrored UPMR database kept up to date by the secure healthcare network at the patient's home medical

organization. The mirrored UPMR can only be changed by the secure healthcare network.
8. A mirrored UPMR for an individual can be available for view by the individual if the home medical organization chooses. This would involve medical organization determined security measures. This disallows anyone to directly access UPMRs in the secure healthcare network through the Internet.
9. A mirrored UPMR will be data belonging to the home medical organization. Many medical organizations today provide patient access to his/her medical information with medical organization determined security, so mirrored UPMR access just extends this capability.
10. Outside medical organization source documents will exist in a mirrored UPMR database but no local source documents, as these can be retrieved through the medical organization EMR system.
11. There will be a research database that includes de-identified UPMR and source document information
12. How will source documents in the research database be de-identified, as some source documents may not identify some fields or be scanned documents?
13. Will biomarker information, for example in procedures, be standardized so population research can be done on it? Is this feasible?
14. Will the list of significant health problems be standardized?
15. How can quality-of-life measurements be added to the UPMR (including longitudinal disease histories in the UPMR) if the individual does not come in for care? Proposed was that the individual send quality-of-life (and sometimes pain) measures to the home medical organization that will record them and update UPMR information the next time the individual comes in for care.
16. Biometric information will be collected at an outside medical organization to allow access to the patient's UPMR at that medical organization. Is that feasible? Biometric information enables a physician at an outside medical organization to see a patient's UPMR

17. How can biometric information be entered?
18. Will medial organizations allow healthcare network retrieval of source documents?
19. Small medical organizations can offload administrative functions (insurance, patient payments, medical personnel payments) to the utility EMR organization. Is this feasible?
20. New software capabilities in EMR systems must be programed for source document retrieval. What would compel the large number of medical organizations to make the necessary changes to enable this retrieval?
21. What would compel medical organizations to periodically review the medications of patients when this may negatively hurt drug companies?
22. What would compel commercial ancillary care systems to interface with the secure healthcare network? Note that pharmacies would work differently in informing the secure healthcare network that a medication was dispensed.
23. Will physicians take responsibility for extended care (the three C's)?
24. Will physicians agree to track significant health problems and initiate and update longitudinal disease histories?
25. Because of a conflict of interest, should a consulting pharmacist be prohibited from selling medications?
26. Can physicians be compelled to follow care plans in cases and episodes of care?
27. How do you get patients to understand quality-of-life measures and get them to input values even if they are not sick?
28. Can patients understand the complexity of sharing genetic information?
29. Who is in control for complicated medical problems that need to be treated at a remote medical organization and perhaps then treated at the patient's home medical organization?
30. Can physicians in rural areas agree to work together?

More broadly,

1. How do you get input and buy-in from the many groups dealing with healthcare? Who pays for this?
2. How do you get the many medical organizations of the world to agree upon a UPMR? Who will pay for implementation, including creation and re-programming of EMR systems?

How will the changes in the way medicine is practiced be agreed upon and accomplished?

# 35. Where to Next?

I have written a Kindle book, *Disruptive Medicine: An Educated Patient's Perspective* (McGuire, 2015), which is an example of a requirements document developed to determine how medicine should change in the future to greatly improve patient care.

My *requirements document* presents the results of a *requirements analysis*, where the requirements analysis goes through the following steps to determine how medicine should be changed: (1) identify how medicine currently functions, functions badly, and could function better; (2) identify how medicine is likely to change in the future; and (3) use this information to determine future best practices and software systems that would improve patient care. Only then should solutions be developed to implement these best practices and systems, as currently existing solutions may not be the best or even good solutions for the future.

A major change in medicine in the future is likely to be combining a patient's medical records from different medical organizations where the patient was seen for care. The current idea on how to do this is EMR system to EMR system interoperability. I think that the requirements analysis would show that that interoperability may not be the best approach to combining a patient's medical information.

To truly identify improvements to medicine, this process of requirements analysis should not be done by one person (as I did in my "Disruptive Medicine" book), but by the medical community, governments, patients, public health, researchers and other interested parties. They should start from scratch in their analysis and determine the best solutions, not necessarily the existing ones!

This book presents my ideas on how medicine should change after I did my own requirements analysis.

# Glossary

**appointment type search:** see "type search."

**accountability:** measuring the performance of a physician or other medical professional in doing a procedure to evaluate the quality of care provided.

**active drugs:** drugs that work before they are metabolized (Cho & Yoon, 2018).

**advance directive:** a document which provides guidance to medical professionals on the patient's care if the patient cannot speak for himself or herself in hypothetical future situations at the end of life.

**ancillary services:** supplemental or diagnostic services provided in support of, or in addition to, care delivered by a primary clinician.

**artificial intelligence (AI):** Artificial intelligence in medicine involves AI making diagnostic or treatment decisions that a physician would normally make based upon an AI engine being trained with data a physician would see to make past decisions together with the corresponding outcomes of each of these past decisions (confirmed diagnoses or treatment results).

**bacteriophage:** a virus that kills a specific type of bacteria (Chhibber et al., 2008).

**big data:** a large data set (e.g., all a patient's source documents) that can computationally reveal patterns, trends, and associations. More specifically big data is used in medicine for predictive modeling and clinical decision support, disease or safety surveillance, public health, and research.

**biomarker:** cellular, biochemical, molecular or genetic characteristic or alteration by which a normal, abnormal, or simply biologic process can be recognized, or monitored (McGuire, 2015).

**biometrics:** an automated way of recognizing a person by physical information such as the person's face, iris, fingerprints, handwriting or voice.

**bookable time:** a time in a schedule when an identified type of appointment can be booked.

**call center:** a group of appointment clerks, advice nurses and advice physicians who make appointments and guide the patient in either seeking medical care or providing self-care.

**capitated medical organization:** a medical organization instead of only getting paid by insurers for fee-for-service, gets paid an amount each month per member to provide comprehensive medical care.

**capsule tear:** a tear to a lens capsule that is a clear, thin transparent membrane that holds the lens within the eye, whether this is the original or replacement lens (Wikipedia, 2023b).

**case:** non-source document medical related information kept for an individual over a significant period of time, even over the individual's lifetime, to ensure care that satisfies the three C's for a specific medical condition or concern.

**catalog of medical services:** a proposed on-line catalog of available medical services, including the geographic location of the service and requirements of a patient to receive the service.

**center of medical expertise:** A medical organization providing very specialized care, being the only one or one of a few such medical organizations providing this care.

**chatbot:** A program to simulate conversations with a user.

**clinical practice guidelines:** recommendations on how to diagnose and treat a medical condition, mainly written for doctors, but also for nurses and other health care professionals (NIH,2020).

**clinical summary:** a summary of medical information for an individual.

**clinical trials**: a very structured set of tests to evaluate new drugs and treatments that are not yet included in clinical practice guidelines, with successful clinical trials possibly resulting in changes to guidelines.

**confirmed diagnosis**: a diagnosis that is confirmed objectively by observations and tests.

**connecting the dots:** looking for events and connections between events in longitudinal disease histories and including biomarkers.

**consistency of care:** the care plan is not inconsistently changed from one encounter to another.

**consultation (or consult):** a physician evaluating a patient at the request of another physician.

**consulting pharmacist**: a pharmacist, rather than selling medications, who will guide a patient and the patient's physician in using, prescribing, changing, curtailing and scheduling medications.

**continuity of care:** the patient comes in for care as necessary; the patient is not forgotten.

**control:** a group used as a standard of comparison for checking the results of an experiment.

**coordination of care:** there is a physician to manage and coordinate care.

**dedicated EMR system:** an EMR system connected to the secure healthcare network used by one medical organization.

**de-identified patient data:** data in which all information identifying patients has been removed (McCallister, 2010).

**DICOM (Digital Imaging and Communications in Medicine):** a recognized digital standard for digitized diagnostic images (Pianykh, 2011).

**differential diagnosis:** a possible diagnosis that, together with other differential diagnoses sharing the same signs or symptoms, can be evaluated objectively by observations and tests to lead toward a confirmed diagnosis.

**disease biomarker:** a biomarker to identify a specific disease.

**disease history:** Either the disease history recorded in a SOAP note, or the shortened name for a longitudinal disease history.

**disease pathways:** changes internal to cells leading to a disease as a result of genetic and environmental factors.

**disruptive medicine:** changing medicine in a dramatic way to greatly improve the way medicine is currently practiced.

**early treatment diseases:** diseases that have the potential of being predicted and treated before there are symptoms that the disease has occurred.

**electronic medical record (EMR) system:** a software system to input medical information and take the place of paper medical records storing this information on a database. An EMR system might interface with other software systems to do ordering and return of results (e.g., prescriptions; clinical laboratory; hospital admission, discharge and transfer; appointments).

**emergency severity index (ESI):** a number used to identify a level of care for an emergency department, where care varies according to the medical conditions the emergency department can handle and the number of types of physicians needed to care for the patient (Gilboy et al., 2012).

**encounter:** a meeting of a patient with medical personnel or a communication between the two.

**epigenetic changes:** changes in the genome not due to changes in bases (i.e., not due to mutations); mechanisms that turn a gene on or off without changing the cell's genetic code.

**episode of care:** non-source document medical related information kept for an individual until an expected outcome is reached to ensure care that satisfies the three C's for a specific medical condition.

**EQ-5D:** a measure of quality of life in terms of disability, with complete disability having a value of 0.0 and no disability having a value of 1.0 (Brooks & Rabin, 2010).

**evidence-based medicine:** a systematic approach to clinical problem solving which allows the integration of the best available research evidence with clinical expertise and patient values (Masic et al., 2008).

**extra time:** a time in a schedule where an appointment can be booked that does not affect bookable time in the schedule.

**fallback position:** either another intervention that can correct a serious side effect of an intervention or a resulting situation that is not totally catastrophic. For example, a fallback position of a knee replacement causing problems is surgery to correct the problem. A fallback position of a surgery on an eye that could cause blindness is that the patient can still see adequately out of his other eye. If there is no fallback position for an intervention, then a physician should have some reluctance in doing the intervention.

**fee-for-service medical organization:** a medical organization that makes their money by charging for each of the medical services and items they provide a patient, as contrasted to a capitated medical organization.

**futures list entry:** search parameters used to book an appointment in the future in a yet-to-be released schedule.

**game plan:** an outline given to a patient's primary physician to treat a complicated problem, identifying possible diagnoses, tests to be done and specialty physicians who could be consulted to resolve the problem.

**gene:** a sequence of bases in the genome that encodes either an RNA or protein molecule, which, together with other genes, forms a basis for traits in a human being, most significantly traits shared with one's parents and ancestors.

**genome:** the sequences of bases within chromosomes, and the DNA within the chromosomes, that occur within the fertilized egg and are carried over to almost every cell in the human body.

**health problem:** one of an individual's recorded medical conditions.

**health psychologist:** "a psychologist who scientifically assists an individual in changing his or her lifestyle to live a healthier life and prevent disease—be the lifestyle change to stop smoking, stop taking drugs, revise a diet, get more exercise, manage stress, or other change. A health psychologist may also assist an individual in how to live with chronic disease" (Taylor, 2015).

**health psychology:** "a field devoted to understanding psychological influences on how people stay healthy, why they become ill, and how they respond when they do get ill" (Taylor, 2015).

**healthcare proxy:** "a document that names someone the patient trusts as the patient's agent to express his/her wishes and make health care decisions if he/she is unable to speak for herself/himself" (Medicare-interactive, 2003).

**HIPAA (the Health Insurance Portability and Accounting Act of 1996):** an act of the United States Congress that identifies restrictions on the availability of a patient's medical information.

**held time:** a time period in a schedule where no appointments can be booked.

**home healthcare worker:** a physician, nurse or other medical worker who provides care for patients in their homes.

**home medical organization:** a medical organization where an individual is normally seen for care.

**"hospital at home":** home hospital care.

**hospice care:** a type of palliative care for patients who are at the end-of-life.

**house call:** a visit by a physician, nurse practitioner or physician assistant to a patient's home.

**ICU (intensive care unit):** a unit of a hospital devoted to patients with severe or life-threatening illnesses or injuries.

**informed consent:** when a healthcare provider explains a medical treatment to a patient to allow the patient to ask questions and accept or deny treatment (healthline, 2023).

**inpatient stay:** in a bed at a hospital or in a hospital at home program.

**interoperability:** "allowing the EMR system in the current medical organization where the patient is being seen to get medical information from the EMR system of the medical organization where the patient is normally seen for care."

**intervention:** The act of intervening, interfering or interceding with the intent of modifying the outcome, with the intervention undertaken to help treat or cure a condition.)

**longitudinal disease history:** a non-source document providing a detailed history of one of a patient's medical conditions over his or her lifetime. In this book this term is shortened to "disease history".

**longevity:** how long a person lives or how long a patient lives after a given intervention or series of interventions or after the beginning of a given medical condition.

**medical alliance:** a group of physicians, nurses and clinics who work together in a rural setting.

**messaging:** the ability for a patient or medical personnel to send and receive back an email to and from a physician with the received email going through a nurse to prioritize the urgency of the response.

**metabolic syndrome:** a combination of visceral obesity, abnormally elevated cholesterol in the blood, an abnormally high blood glucose level, and hypertension.

**mirrored UPMR database:** a copy of the patient's UPMR kept for a patient at the patient's home medical organization that is kept up to date by the UPMR. It can be used for display to the patient and studies using the research database.

**mutation:** changes in bases in the genome (DNA) of a cell that occur over time, for example, errors that randomly occur when cells divide.

**NANDA (North American Nursing Diagnosis Association):** an association that identifies nursing diagnoses for inpatients and associated interventions to mitigate each nursing diagnosis.

**non-bookable time:** a time in a schedule where there are no appointments booked, either time seeing patients or not seeing patients.

**nursing diagnosis:** a possible situation for an inpatient that could cause an adverse health condition (e.g., risk of falling, risk of pressure ulcer) for which interventions could be taken to mitigate the adverse condition (e.g., keep the room free of clutter, reposition the patient in bed every 2 hours).

**outcome:** ways of measuring a patient's health, especially after a medical intervention

**outside medical organization referral:** a referral to a physician not at a patient's home medical organization. This is important to distinguish from a referral inside the patient's home medical organization as the secure healthcare network will need to allow the referred-to physician to have access to the patient's medical information in the secure healthcare network in order to process the referral.

**overall biomarker:** a biomarker commonly recorded during many medical visits (e.g., temperature, blood pressure, oxygen saturation).

**overall case:** a case for a patient who is a high utilizer of services that covers all of the patient's medical conditions and is managed by a clinical social worker rather than a physician.

**outpatient visit:** a face-to-face or telehealth meeting of a patient with a physician or other healthcare professional. This includes emergency department visits.

**palliative care:** care focusing on quality of life rather than cure.

**patient advocate:** a person who serves as a liaison between a patient and that patient's healthcare providers to improve or maintain a high quality of healthcare for the patient.

**pattern matching:** determining the diagnosis for a patient based upon previous patients presenting with the same symptoms, assuming the patient is similar to those other patients.

**personal health goals (goals):** a patient's goals in life that could be used to determine appropriate medical care.

**physician analyst:** a technology-oriented physician who will work closely together with a physician consultant to analyze complicated medical problems, with the physician analyst spending much of the time doing data analysis and consulting with specialty physicians to do research on the medical problem. This may result in the physician analyst identifying clinical trials that might be appropriate for the patient. A physician analyst might also have responsibility for doing accountability analyses for the medical organization medical personnel.

**physician consultant:** a physician who will work closely together with a physician analyst to analyze complicated medical problems, with the physician consultant spending most of the time meeting with the patient.

**personalized medicine:** an old term for precision medicine as it is medicine applied to a smaller group of patients, not just for the one patient. See precision medicine.

**POLST (Provider Orders for Life-Sustaining Treatment): a medical** order developed by a physician talking to the patient based upon the current condition of the patient to provide guidance to medical professionals on the patient's care if the patient cannot speak for himself or herself.

**precision medicine**: a treatment more tailored to the patient due to medicine becoming more complicated, especially due to diagnosis at the cellular level besides the tissue level, resulting in what was viewed as one disease in the past becoming many different ones now (e.g., estrogen positive or negative breast cancer rather than simply breast cancer).

**predictive biomarkers:** biomarkers collected prior to an intervention that could predict the outcomes of the intervention, where the outcomes could later be determined by comparing the pre-intervention biomarkers to the results biomarkers.

**pre-intervention biomarkers:** biomarkers that should be collected prior to an intervention that can later be compared against the results biomarkers to determine the outcomes of the intervention.

**pressure ulcer:** "injury to skin and underlying tissue resulting from prolonged pressure on the skin" (Mayo Clinic, 2023). Pressure ulcers are also called "pressure sores" or "bedsores".

**procedure:** an intervention requiring specialized expertise. Examples are doing a surgery or interpreting a mammogram for breast cancer.

**prodrugs:** drugs that work after they are metabolized (Cho & Yoon, 2018).

**QALY (quality of life years):** a way of both measuring quality of life and longevity.

**quality of life:** a measure of an individual's disabilities, if any together with personal factors affecting the attitude of the individual.

**randomized control study:** a research study based upon a hypothesis where individuals are randomly put into two groups, one group undergoing what is to be researched testing the hypothesis and the other being put into a control group where they think they are part of the research group but are not. This type of study minimizes researcher bias in that individuals will not be selected for the research group that are more likely to produce more favorable results for the researcher. The study is also done so the researcher cannot favor one group over the other.

**receptor:** proteins either on the surface of a cell or internal to a cell which can bind with hormones, neurotransmitters, drugs, toxins, viruses or microbes which can result in a change in the activity of the cell, including allowing in molecules or viruses into the cell.

**requirements document:** a document describing how a software system would function in all areas of an organization or in an industry.

**referral:** either a request that the referred-to physician provide consultation advice to the referring physician or that the referred-to physician set up a meeting with the patient.

**remote healthcare worker:** a physician or nurse or other healthcare worker who works from his or her home and uses telehealth or visits patients in their homes, seldom going to a medical facility.

**remote medical organization:** a medical organization that is not a patient's home medical organization.

**results biomarkers:** biomarkers that can be measured after an intervention that identify the results (outcomes) of the intervention.

**retina:** "a light-sensitive layer of tissue that forms an inner coat of the eye" (Wikipedia, 2023d).

**retinal detachment:** "a disorder of the eye where the retina separates from the layer underneath" (Wikipedia, 2023e).

**roadmap:** a plan of care in the form of a string of the complaint, differential diagnoses, tests and procedures which could lead to a confirmed diagnosis for a complicated medical condition.

**secure healthcare network:** software and an associated database that connects EMR systems, enabling the controlled display of a patient's combined medical information gathered from all medical organizations where the patient received care.

**schedule release:** making schedules for a department or subdepartment within a date range available for booking.

**sepsis:** a potentially life-threatening condition resulting from the presence of live harmful organisms in the blood or other tissues and the body's response to their presence, potentially leading to malfunctioning of various organs.

**self-care checklist:** a list of things an individual should do to avoid medical problems and information on when the individual should come in for medical care.

**side effects:** unintended outcomes of an intervention.

**significant health problem:** a standardized list of health problems to be tracked for all patients.

**SOAP note:** the most common form of textual medical record with SOAP standing for subjective, objective, assessment and plan parts of the SOAP note.

**source documents:** encounter and consult based medical records created as part of an encounter or consult that must be signed off and cannot be changed once signed off.

**standard of care:** a legal term for medicine meaning "the level and type of care that a reasonably competent and skilled health care professional, with a similar background and in the same medical community, would have provided under the circumstances that led to the alleged malpractice" (Nolo, 2023).

**telehealth:** the communication between healthcare workers and a patient or patient advocate via telephone or teleconferencing for the care of the patient.

**telehealth consultation:** a physician or other provider consulting with a patient and/or patient advocate via telehealth or observing a patient via telehealth during a hospital at home stay. A telehealth communication can constitute a telehealth encounter or occur as part of a hospital at home stay.

**telehealth encounter:** an outpatient encounter via telehealth of a patient with a physician or other medical provider.

**the three C's:** three possible problems with encounter-based medical care: coordination of care, continuity of care, and consistency of care.

**time search:** a search for bookable time in a schedule of a length identified by an appointment type that would be used to book the appointment.

**type search:** a search for a bookable time in a schedule that enables booking an appointment with an identified appointment type.

**utility EMR system:** an EMR system connected to the secure healthcare network used by more than one medical organization.

**virtual facility:** a way a large medical organization could provide care in an area without a large medical facility being there.

**"virtual hospital":** a situation where a large portion of inpatient care is provided by "hospital at home." (Note that this definition differs from definitions currently used by some medical organizations.)

**virtual organization:** a situation where one physician supervises other physicians in the care of a patient where this relationship applies just for this patient. This often occurs during hospital stays, especially when there is an attending physician who recruits specialty physicians to provide care for the patient.

ENVISIONING MEDICINE IN THE FUTURE

# References

Ahuja A. S. (2019). The impact of artificial intelligence in medicine on the future role of the physician. *PeerJ, 7*, e7702. https://doi.org/10.7717/peerj.7702

AI Brew. (2025). UCSF Study Shows AI Can Draft Hospital Discharge Summaries, Saving Clinicians Time. AI Brew News. Retrieved August 3, 2025 from https://aibrew.news/articles/ucsf-study-shows-ai-can-draft-hospital-discharge-summaries-saving-clinicians-time

Alberti, K., Zimmet, P., & Shaw, J. (2005). The metabolic syndrome—a new worldwide definition. *The Lancet, 366*(9491), 4. .\

ANKE. (2023). CT scan mobile radiology room. CT scan mobile radiology room.

Association of American Medical Colleges. (2023, March 29, 2023). AAMC Supports Resident Physician Shortage Reduction Act of 2023 https://www.aamc.org/news/press-releases/aamc-supports-resident-physician-shortage-reduction-act-2023#:~:text=According%20to%20AAMC%20data%2C%20the, demand%20for%20physicians%20 outpacing%20supply

Apple. (2024). *Share your AF History*. Apple. https://support.apple.com/en-ie/HT212214#:~:text=Apple%20Watch%20cannot%20detect%20a,instance%20of%20your%20irregular%20rhythm

Belle, A., Thiagarajan, R., Soroushmehr, S. M. R., Navidi, F., Beard, D. A., & Najarian, K. (2015). Big Data Analytics in Healthcare. BioMed Research International, 2015, 370194. https://doi.org/10.1155/2015/370194

Bennett, J., Sandford, D., Kandel, E., Rose, C., Schwarz, S., Shatz, C., & Zrenner, E. (Writers) & E. Kandel (Director). (2014). Charlie Rose Brain Series: Blindness. In Charlie Rose Brain Series: Blindness.

Blackburn, E., & Epel, E. (2017). The Telomere Effect: A Revolutionary Approach to Living Younger, Healthier, Longer. Grand Central Publishing.

Brett, MS. (2024). Long-Term Outcomes After False-Positive Mammography Results. *Journal Watch*, *44*(5), 43-44.

Brooks, R., & Rabin, R. (2010). The Measurement and Valuation of Health Status Using EQ-5D: A European Perspective: Springer.

Brown, T. (2019, April 27, 2019). How to Mke Doctors Think About Death, Opinion. New York Times.Centers-for-Disease-Control-and-Prevention. (2022). Prediabetes – Your Chance to Prevent Type 2 Diabetes. https://www.cdc.gov/diabetes/basics/prediabetes.html

Buchanan B. G., Shortliffe E. H. (1984). Rule-Based Expert Systems: The MYCIN Experiments of the Stanford Heuristic Programming Project. Addison Wesley.

Buckley, L. (2016). Bates' Guide to Physical Examination and History Taking: Wolters Kluwer.

Chan, F. M., Mathur, R., Ku, J. J. K., Chen, C., Chan, S.-P., Yong, V. S. H., & Eong, K.-G. A. (2003). Short-term outcomes in eyes with posterior capsule rupture during cataract surgery. Journal of Cataract & Refractive Surgery, 29(3), 5

Chhibber, S., Kaur, S., & Kumari, S. (2008). Therapeutic potential of bacteriophage in treating Klebsiella pneumoniae B5055-mediated lobar pneumonia in mice. Jouranl of Medical Microbiology, 57(12), 6.

Cho S., & Yoon, Y. R. (2018). Understanding the pharmacokinetics of prodrug and metabolite. Translational and clinical pharmacology, 26(1), 1–5. https://doi.org/10.12793/tcp.2018.26.1.1

Cimons, M. (2024). A blood test to detect cancer? Some patients are using them already. (April 16, 2024 ). https://www.washingtonpost.com/wellness/interactive/2024/cancer-blood-test-screening/

CMS. (2023). Find a patient advocate. Centers for Medicare & Medicaid Services. https://www.cms.gov/medical-bill-rights/help/guides/patient-advocate

Doudna, J., & Charpentier, E. (2014). The new frontier of genome engineering with CRISPR-Cas9. Science, 346(6213)

Finch, J. (2023). point-to point. www.finchmagician.com/video-conferencing/point-to-point

Centers for Disease Control and Prevention. (2022). Prediabetes – Your Chance to Prevent Type 2 Diabetes. https://www.cdc.gov/diabetes/basics/prediabetes.html

Dall, T., Reynolds, R., Chakrabarti, R., Ruttinger, C., Zarek, P., & Parker, O. (2024). The Complexities of Physician Supply and Demand: Projections From 2021 to 2036. https://www.aamc.org/media/75236/download

Desaia, P., Minassianb, D. C., & Reidy, A. (1999). National cataract surgery survey 1997–8: a report of the results of the clinical outcomes. British Journal of Ophthalmology, 83(12)

Dressler, D. (2019). Hospital at Home Is Supported by a Randomized Trial. NEJM Journal Watch(December 19, 2019)

Freschi, C., Ferrari, V., Melfi, F., Ferrari, M., Mosca, F., & Cuschieri, A. (2013). Technical Review of the da Vinci Surgical Telemanipulator. The international journal of medical robotics + computer assisted surgery : *MRCAS*, *9*(4), 396–406. https://doi.org/10.1002/rcs.1468

Gawande, A. (2003). Being Mortal: Medicine and What Matters in the End. New York: Metropolitan Books.

Gawande, A. (2009). The Checklist Manifesto: How to Get Things Right. New York Metropolitan Books.

Goodman, A. (2007). Human Body: How We Fail, How We Heal. Great Courses. Chantilly, Virginia: The Teaching Company.

Gordon, D. (2022). The Return Of House Calls? New Survey Reveals Health Leaders' Outlook On Care At Home. https://www.forbes.com/sites/debgordon/2022/12/13/the-return-of-house-calls-new survey-reveals-health-leaders-outlook-on-care-at-home/?sh=33814432d11e

GRAIL. (2024). Pathfinder 2 Study. https://grail.com/clinical-studies/pathfinder-2-study/

Health Insurance Portability and Accountability Act of 1996, H.R. 3103 (1996).

healthline. (2023). What You Need to Know About Informed Consent. healthline. https://www.healthline.com/health/informed-consent

Institutional Review Board. (2003). Definition of De-Identified Data. John Hopkins Medicine. https://www.hopkinsmedicine.org/institutional_review_board/hipaa_research/de_identified_da ta.html

Kandel, E., & Rose, C. (Writers) & E. Kandel & C. Rose (Directors). (2012). Charlie Rose Brain Series 2: Alzheimers Disease. In Charlie Rose Brain Series 2: Public Broadcasting Service.

Kelm, D. J., Perrin, J. T., Cartin-Ceba, R., Gajic, O., Schenck, L., & Kennedy, C. C. (2015). Fluid overload in patients with severe sepsis and septic shock treated with early goal-directed therapy is associated with increased acute need for fluid-related medical interventions and hospital death. Shock (Augusta, Ga.), 43(1), 68–73.

KFF. (2023). Preventive Services Covered by Private Health Plans under the Affordable Care Act. https://www.kff.org/report-section/preventive-service-tracker-immunizations/

Knight, J. (2022). The Healthcare Super-utilizer and the United States of Healthcare. https://medcitynews.com/2022/09/the-healthcare-super-utilizer-and-the-united-states-of healthcare/

Lawrence, D. (2003). From Chaos To Care: The Promise Of Team-based Medicine. Da Capo Press.

Littman, M. L. (2020). Introduction to Machine Learning. Chantilly, VA, The Teaching Company.

Makary, M. (2013). Unaccountable: What Hospitals Won't Tell You and How Transparency Can Revolutionize Health Care. Bloomsbury Press.

Masic, I., Miokovic, M., Muhamedagic, B. (2008). Evidence Based Medicine – New Approaches and Challenges. Acta Inform Med., 16(4), 219–225

Mayo Clinic. (2023). Bed sores (pressure ulcers). Mayo Foundation. https://www.mayoclinic.org/diseases-conditions/bed-sores/symptoms causes/syc-20355893

McCallister, E. (2010). Guide to Protecting the Confidentiality of Personally Identifiable Information (PII).

McFarland, G. K., & McFarlane, E. A. (1997). Nursing Diagnosis & Intervention: Planning for Patient Care (No. 974): Mosby Incorporated.

McGuire, M. R. (2015). Disruptive Medicine: An Educated Patient's Perspective. McGuire Publishing.

Mold, J. W. (2017). Achieving Your Personal Health Goals: A Patient's Guide. Englewood Cliffs, NJ: Full Court Press

Montie, E. (2023). Elon Musk's xAI Announces New Data Center: Where Do A.I. Giants Store Their Data?

National Library of Science. (2023). What Is the Difference Between Precision Medicine and Personalized Medicine? What About Pharmacogenomics? https://medlineplus.gov/genetics/understanding/precisionmedicine/precisionvspersonalized/

NIH. (2020). What Are Clinical Practice Guidelines? NIH National Library of Medicine. https://www.ncbi.nlm.nih.gov/books/NBK390308/

Novak, M. (2012). Predictions From The Father of Science Fiction. Smithsonian Magazine. https://www.smithsonianmag.com/history/predictions-from-the-father-of-science-fiction 61256664/

Olsen, T., & Jeppesen, P. (2012). The Incidence of Retinal Detachment After Cataract Surgery. The Open Ophthalmology Journal, 12(6), 4.

Onisko A., T. A., Druzdzel M.J. (2015). Prediction and Prognosis of Health and Disease. In L. P. Hommersom A. (Ed.), Foundations of Biomedical Knowledge Representation. Lecture Notes in Computer Science (Vol. 9521, pp. 181-188): Springer.

Park, A. (2023). Scientists Have Reached a Key Milestone in Learning How to Reverse Aging. *Time*. https://time.com/6246864/reverse-aging-scientists-discover-milestone/

Parsons, A. S. (2020). Inappropriate Medications in Older Adults at Discharge. NEJM Journal Watch(June 25, 2020). https://www.jwatch.org/na51891/2020/06/25/inappropriate-medications-older adults-discharge

PBS. (2024). Cancer Detectives.

Pearl, R. (2025). Will Your Next Surgeon Be a Robot?. https://www.forbes.com/sites/robertpearl/2025/12/01/will-your-next-surgeon-be-a-robot/

Pearl, R. (2024). ChatGPT, MD: How AI-Empowered Patients & Doctors Can Take Back Control of American Medicine.

Pearl, R. (2017). Mistreated: Why We Think We're Getting Good Health Care—and Why We're Usually Wrong. Public Affairs.

Pepplinkhuizen, S., Hoeksema, W. F., van der Stuijt, W., van Steijn, N. J., Winter, M. M., Wilde, A. A. M., Smeding, L., & Knops, R. E. (2022). Accuracy and clinical relevance of the single-lead Apple Watch electrocardiogram to identify atrial fibrillation. *Cardiovascular digital health journal*, *3*(6 Suppl), S17–S22. https://doi.org/10.1016/j.cvdhj.2022.10.004

Pianykh, O. S. (2012). Digital Imaging Imaging and Co"unication in Medicine (DICOM): A Pratical Introduction and Survival Guide. Springer Nature.

Podder, V., Lew, V., & Ghassemzadeh, S. (2023). SOAP Notes. StatPearls Publishing.

Potter, j. (2021). Is Suicide the Unforgivable Sin? Understanding Suicide, Stigma, and Salvation through Two Christian Perspectives. Religion, 12(11), 987.

Prendiville, W., Cullimore, J., & Norman, S. (1989). Large loop excision of the transformation ) (LLETZ). A new method of management for women with cervical intraepithelial neoplasia. *British journal of obstetrics and gynaecology*, *96*(9), 1054–1060. https://doi.org/10.1111/j.1471-0528.1989.tb03380.x

Pugle, M. (2019). *Want to Lower Your Sodium Intake? Consider Potassium Chloride Instead of Salt*. Health News. https://www.healthline.com/health-news/what-is-potassium-chloride-and-why-you-may-want-to-replace-salt-with-it

Quora. (2023). Can a Nurse Perform a Physical Exam? quora.
    https://www.quora.com/Can-a-nurse perform-a-physical-exam
Sapolsky, R. (2010). Stress and Your Body. The Great Courses.
Smith, K. (2011). BRCA Mutation Testing in Determining Breast Cancer
    Therapy. Cancer Journal, 7(6), 8
Sulakvelidze, A., Alavidze, Z., & J. Glenn Morris, J. (2001). Bacteriophage
    Therapy. Antimicrobial Agents and Chemotherapy, 45(3), 11.
Swinscow, T. D. V. (1997). Populations and samples. In Statistics at
    Square One. BMJ Publishing Group.
    https://www.bmj.com/about-bmj/resources-
    readers/publications/statistics-square-one/3 populations-and-
    samples
Taylor, S. E. (2015). Health Psychology. New York: McGraw Hill
    Education.
University of California/San Francisco. (2015). Telemedicine Assessment
    and Consultation Team (TACT): Caring for Individuals with
    Complex Developmental Disabilities in Rural Northern
    California San Francisco.
    https://www.uctv.tv/shows/Telemedicine-Assessment-and-
    Consultation-Team-TACT-Caring-for Individuals-with-Complex-
    Developmental-Disabilities-in-Rural-Northern-California-28909
Vulin, M., Magušić, L., Metzger, A. M., Muller, A., Drenjančević, I., Jukić,
    I., Šijanović, S., Lukić, M., Stanojević, L., Davidović Cvetko, E.,
    & Stupin, A. (2022). Sodium-to-Potassium Ratio as an Indicator
    of Diet Quality in Healthy Pregnant Women. *Nutrients*, *14*(23),
    5052. https://doi.org/10.3390/nu14235052
Winawer, N. (2018). Can We Safely Discharge Patients Home Directly
    from the ICU? NEJM Journal Watch(August 30, 2018).
Wikipedia. (2023a). Capsule of lens. In.
Wikipedia (2023b). Capsule tear. In.
Wikipedia (2023c). House Call. In.
Wikipedia. (2023c). Retina. In.
Wikipedia. (2023c). Retinal Detachment. In.
Winawer, N. (2018). Can We Safely Discharge Patients Home Directly
    from the ICU? NEJM Journal Watch(August 30, 2018).

Yang, J. H., Petty, C. A., Dixon-McDougall, T., Lopez, M. V., Tyshkovskiy, A., Maybury-Lewis, S., Tian, X., Ibrahim, N., Chen, Z., Griffin, P. T., Arnold, M., Li, J., Martinez, O. A., Behn, A., Rogers-Hammond, R., Angeli, S., Gladyshev, V. N., & Sinclair, D. A. (2023). Chemically induced reprogramming to reverse cellular aging. *Aging, 15*(13), 5966–5989. https://doi.org/10.18632/aging.204896

Wojtara, M., Rana, E., Rahman, T., Khanna, P., & Singh, H. (2023). Artificial intelligence in rare disease diagnosis and treatment. *Clinical and translational science, 16*(11), 2106–2111. https://doi.org/10.1111/cts.13619

Young, J. (2024). AI Will Help the World's Top Hospital CEOs Transform Health Care. https://www.newsweek.com/2024/03/15/how-ai-will-help-worlds-top-hospital-ceos-transform-health-care-1872947.html

Zare, M., Javadi, M. h.-A., Einollahi, B., Baradaran-Rafii, A.-R., Feizi, S., & Kiavash, V. (2009). Risk Factors for Posterior Capsule Rupture and and Vitreous Loss during Phacoemulsification. Journal of Ophthalmic & Vision Research, 4(4), 5.

www.ingramcontent.com/pod-product-compliance
Lightning Source LLC
Chambersburg PA
CBHW031630210526
45464CB00004B/1834